D0412939

I'm Too Hot Now

UHB TRUST LIBRARY
WITHDRAWN FROM STOCK

To
David Haslam,
because he is a fine doctor and a passionate advocate for general practice, and was, from 2001 to 2004, an inspiring Chairman of Council of the Royal College of General Practitioners. But mainly because I admire him as a person and prize him as a friend.

I'm Too Hot Now

Themes and variations from general practice

Roger Neighbour

MA, DSc, FRCP, PRCGP

Foreword by

Professor Carol Black CBE

President
Royal College of Physicians

Radcliffe Publishing
Oxford • Seattle

Radcliffe Publishing Ltd
18 Marcham Road
Abingdon
Oxon OX14 1AA
United Kingdom

www.radcliffe-oxford.com
Electronic catalogue and worldwide online ordering facility.

© 2005 Roger Neighbour

All rights reserved. No part of this publication may be reproduced, stored in
a retrieval system or transmitted, in any form or by any means, electronic, mech-
anical, photocopying, recording or otherwise without the prior permission of the
copyright owner.

British Library Cataloguing in Publication Data

A catalogue record for this book is available from the British Library.

ISBN 1 85775 654 1

Typeset by Aarontype Ltd, Easton, Bristol
Printed and bound by TJ International Ltd, Padstow, Cornwall

Contents

Foreword

I'm Too Hot Now is a collection of reviews, lectures, commentaries, and speculations produced by Dr Roger Neighbour over the past 15 years. It is a captivating journey through the landscape of general practice. It offers a landscape drawn with a fresh and sharp eye. Dr Neighbour brings a keen, impatient, often iconoclastic, yet almost always warm and generous imagination to size up the world he lives in. He gives the reader a uniquely personal view on many themes, reaching far beyond the familiar territory of practice yet almost always pertinent to it. The passion and reflective curiosity that first drew him to medicine have not wavered with the realities of service, and he has little time for those who seem not to accept or perhaps even wish to understand the special qualities of the immensely human encounters that can make general practice the most rewarding of all the specialties.

He brings a light touch to serious matters; stuffed with wisdom and garnished with humour, sour only when called for. He is not afraid to question the earnest academic footings that give General Practice the standing it enjoys today and mark its differences from the procedure driven specialties that more readily capture media and public attention.

This book is not just for doctors: thoughtful patients, the public and politicians will find time for it too. Many of the situations and experiences Dr Neighbour describes and draws on will be familiar to these people, but his insights and questioning will be new.

Professor Carol Black CBE
President, Royal College of Physicians
January 2005

About the author

From 1974 to 2003, Roger Neighbour was a general practitioner in Abbots Langley, Hertfordshire. He was a trainer for many years, and course organiser of the Watford VTS from 1979 to 1986, being awarded the inaugural Fellowship of the Association of Course Organisers in 1988. His interest in the relationship between doctor and patient, and that between teacher and learner, emerged from reading experimental psychology at Cambridge University; a six-year period in a Balint group; participation in a Nuffield Course run by the late Paul Freeling; training in experiential psychotherapy at Surrey University; and in Ericksonian hypnosis in Phoenix, Arizona. An examiner for the MRCGP examination for 20 years from 1984, he was Convenor of the Panel of Examiners from 1997 to 2002. In 2003 he was elected to the Presidency of the Royal College of General Practitioners.

Roger Neighbour has published numerous columns, reviews, papers and book chapters on vocational training and assessment; the MRCGP examination; problem-solving and decision-making; medical current affairs; and medico-philosophical issues. A second edition of his book *The Inner Consultation* (reprinted nine times since its publication in 1987) is published by Radcliffe Publishing as a companion to *The Inner Apprentice*. In it, he explores the skills GPs need if they are to manage their central activity – consulting – effectively.

Acknowledgements

I'm enormously grateful to Carol Black, President of the Royal College of Physicians, for contributing the foreword to this anthology. Forewords are not mere formalities; the foreword writer actually has to *read* the text, which is no small intrusion into the life of a busy person. And the author, knowing this, has to respect her opinion enough to risk asking for it. Although I've known Carol only a short time, she has my respect in spades. As the head of a medical Royal College, she exemplifies how the interests of her professional constituency and those of the wider community of patients can be harmonised. I was nervous of asking her, but so pleased that I did. Thank you, Carol.

To Andrew Bax and the team at Radcliffe Publishing — Gillian, Jamie, Lisa, Nicola, Iti, Suse — I want to say a different kind of 'thank you'. They are a competent and friendly crew. Andrew in particular has championed general practice publishing way beyond the usual bounds of commercial prudence. But what I feel for the Radcliffe people is a kind of accumulated warmth tinged with relief, such as one might feel when, in middle age, one sees one's parents indulging one's child (or manuscript) with grandparental good humour. Authors thrive on vanity, but depend on encouragement. Radcliffe understand this.

Over the years, numerous friends have supported me more than they may have realised at the time. Declan Dwyer, the first editor of the 'Green Journal', allowed me to build a platform as a reviewer of books. His successor, John Pitts, bravely forbore to pull some of my more eccentric pieces. Alec Logan, editor of the *Back Pages* of the *British Journal of General Practice*, helped temper my adolescent cynicism with a necessary pride in the writer's craft. David Jewell, editor of the *BJGP*, kindly gave permission for the *Back Pages* pieces to be included in this book.

Much of my analysis of what is good and bad about British general practice took shape while I was Convenor of the MRCGP examination. This is no coincidence. To be an MRCGP examiner is to test one's opinions against some of the keenest minds in the country. Peter Tate in particular has been both a catalyst and a friend, as have Tom Dastur and his colleagues in the RCGP's Examination Department.

I'm grateful to Brian Newbould, Emeritus Professor of Music at the University of Hull, for his interest in my Schubert hypothesis, set out in Chapter 12, and to Ashgate Publishing Limited for permission to reproduce it.

The 'penguin' cartoon on the cover is by William Spring, and was published in *Punch* magazine. I liked it so much that I bought the original. *Punch* is now sadly defunct, and I've not been able to trace Mr Spring to secure his permission to reproduce his image. But I hope he won't mind.

Most of all, however, I want to thank various readers who over the years were kind enough, or rash enough, to suggest a collection such as this. They have only themselves to blame.

Disclaimer

The opinions in this book are my own personal ones. More to the point, most of the pieces in it were written before I was elected in 2003 to the Presidency of the Royal College of General Practitioners, an organisation whose purpose and values I wholeheartedly support. Until then, I thought that constructive criticism of the College was the highest form of loyalty to it. But now, having taken up office, I realise that trying to do something positive on its behalf is better than sniping from the safety of print. I'm fortunate to have had the opportunity to do both.

So: the views expressed in these pages are, or were, my own. They may not always be the views or policies of the Royal College of General Practitioners.

1

Introduction

Dissatisfaction, as the cartoon on the cover shows, is the natural state of penguins. And of mankind.

The Buddha reckoned that dissatisfaction springs from always wanting things to be other than they are. (*Human* dissatisfaction, that is; they didn't have penguins in 600 BC.) We human beings want the things we dislike to hurry up and change, while the things we like we want to stay permanently the same. Some hope. The world obstinately carries on being the way it is whether we like it or not, and it changes in its own good time, not ours. We can't rely on reversing the natural order to make ourselves happier.

So what's the answer? The aforesaid Buddha favoured abolishing the sense of a personal self that does the liking and disliking. 'The great way is not difficult,' runs a Zen text, 'it only avoids picking and choosing.'[1] Ah, but how? It's not that easy. The Buddhist curriculum is, in effect, a programme of lifelong learning, with modules covering insight, determination, probity, self-awareness and meditation. It is not given to many – certainly not to me – to stay the course to the point when the 'self that does the suffering' falls away in enlightenment. But in three decades of erratic Zen practice I've had enough tantalising glimpses of what selflessness might be like to be pretty sure the Buddhist cure for dissatisfaction is a real-time possibility. A possibility, but a tough one: practising Buddhism is like sending your ego to boot camp.

By contrast, we in the third millennium regard a strong sense of personal identity not as the obstacle to contentment, but the prize for pursuing it. We have *other* remedies for our dissatisfaction, whole industries whose purpose is to divert us from the human predicament. Having doctors is one way of making ourselves feel better. *Being* a doctor is another. Although not himself a medical man, Ralph Waldo Emerson[2] understood why. 'It is one of the most beautiful compensations of this life,' he observed, 'that no man can sincerely try to help another without helping himself.' Sigmund Freud would probably have put cause and effect the other way round. 'No one,' he might have claimed, 'can defend against neurotic

---

[1] *On faith in the heart*, by Sosan, third Chinese Zen patriarch, roughly contemporary with Christ. It begins:

> The Great Way is not difficult, it only avoids picking and choosing.
> When there is neither hate nor lust, it shines forth in full radiance.
> A hair's breadth of faltering from it, and heaven and earth are set apart.
> If you want to behold it directly, cease from having opinions about it.
> To set up what you want against what you *don't* want – that is the disease of the heart.

[2] American lecturer, essayist and poet, 1803–1882.

impulses without either harming or helping someone else.' From here, it is a straight run to the introspective Balintian tradition in British general practice, with its concepts of 'the doctor as drug' and the doctor's 'apostolic function'[3]. And if we give the theme a further confessional twist, we arrive at 'the wounded healer'[4] – the doctor who is effective because of, not in spite of, his or her psychological baggage. An acknowledgement of frailty can earn a doctor more therapeutic privileges in the patient's own inner world than a façade of superhuman infallibility.

If a career in medicine provides an acceptable, even honourable, way of sublimating the inner demons, so does writing. Most writing, from the greatest classic to the driest academic paper, makes an immodest pitch for the reader's approval. If only people would see things *my* way, the author usually seems to be saying, the world would be a better place – or at least one better understood. For some writers, the desk is a pulpit. Others treat it more like a confessional – and one fitted with a loudspeaker, broadcasting private intimacies to a prurient world. Else it's a mountain top, whence so spectacular a view across the human landscape is gained that one can only gasp, 'Just look at that.'

I suspect writing releases the same habit-forming endorphins in the brain as jogging. Any writer who has had work published – even if it's only 'CLEEN ME' scrawled on the back of a dirty white van – will know the addictive potential of authorship. The trouble is, the business of writing is an effort. As a way of getting other people to sit up and pay attention, streaking is quicker. How odd, therefore, that so many doctors are drawn to commit acts of self-expression – we self-same doctors who in the course of doing the day job endlessly complain about the paperwork! Maybe writers and doctors alike are, to some extent and at some deep level, damaged goods; and the writer-doctor, presumably, double-damaged.

* * *

Whoa! This is getting too heavy. After all, all I'm trying to do is apologise for the cheek of collecting assorted pieces of journalism from the last fifteen years, and passing them off as book-worthy. You're entitled to some explanation.

After my first book, *The inner consultation*, came out in 1987, followed five years later by *The inner apprentice*, lots of nice things started to happen. Nice people said nice things. I got asked to meet more nice people, do nice things, talk to nice groups, teach on nice courses, go to nice places. It was – well, more than nice. It was flattering. More than flattery, it was job creation.

In the spring of 1990, Radcliffe Medical Press, under its generous proprietor Andrew Bax, launched a thrice-yearly journal, *Postgraduate Education for General Practice*. Over the years, and in response to changes of wind direction in medical education and political correctness, it has regularly upgraded its name: to *Education for General Practice* in 1994, and *Education for Primary Care* in 2001. Increasingly successful, it now comes out quarterly, is thicker, and is known affectionately by everyone in the 'friends reunited' world of medical education as 'the Green Journal'. The Green Journal's first Editor was Declan Dwyer, who achieved notoriety as the Darth Vader of the MRCGP examination through his pioneering work on the Critical Reading Question. Declan asked me, in that 'resistance is useless' voice of his, if I would take on the book review section.

---

[3] Balint M (1957) *The doctor, his patient and the illness*. Pitman, London.
[4] Bennett G (1987) *The wound and the doctor*. Secker & Warburg, London.

'Okay', I said, with all the reluctance of an alcoholic asked to help finish off the sherry. 'Books', I wrote in my first column (and I still believe it, even in these multimedia and internet days), 'remain the educational medium consistently voted "most likely to succeed" since 1445.' 'The Journal's book review section,' I promised, 'will scan the printed universe not only for new stars but also for established books worth coming back to, and for books from unexpected quarters with lessons for our professional development.'

Initially I got my friends to write the reviews. I just acted as editor, i.e. sent them threatening letters, and crossed their names one by one off a dwindling list of the not-yet-lumbered. But I quickly decided the monkey could have a better time than the organ grinder; commissioning reviews wasn't as much fun as writing them oneself. I love books: I love them not just for their content, but also for the physical objects they are. I love the heft of them, their smell, the rustle and flick as pages turn. I also love the subtle snobbery of point size, margin width, paper finish; the champagne socialism of a sans serif font and the authority of Times Roman. Not least, I love the effort of authorship that has gone into even the least ambitious or commendable volume. For that reason, I determined never to review a book I thought was not worth buying; better a book ignored than one disparaged.

That said, as I got into my stride, I found myself writing critiques not just of the books, but also of their context, their competition, and sometimes – I confess it – their authors. Reviews *of* books became essays *about* them. My column's by-line evolved from *Book reviews, edited by* ... to *Books*, and finally to *Neighbour on books*. Nice people said nice things. It was flattering. More than flattery, it was hubris.

In 1998 I answered an advert from a national television production company which was recruiting writers for a new soap they were planning, to be set in a GP surgery. They invited me to join their small team of writers developing pilot scripts. Thinking this was advancement, I resigned from my regular Green Journal slot.

The professionals I met on the project were hugely impressive. Some of the other writers were household names, regularly credited on *EastEnders*. Everyone on the production team had put in weeks of research on primary care and the NHS. But we struggled with what remains the hardest problem in dramatising general practice – how to show its subtlety without distorting its truth. The dramas of general practice are usually low-impact affairs: no blue lights, not much blood, few screams, deaths a rarity. Granted, the stories told in the consulting room can be complex and poignant, with life and happiness often at stake. But in the consulting room things by and large are spoken about, not acted, in 10-minute scenes with the actors sitting down, most of the excitement happening off stage and out of time-frame. Ours tend to be narratives in the E M Forster mould, understated and multilayered, not the rollicking good yarns of *Casualty* and *ER*. Gradually it sank in that general practice might make good fiction, but not good four-nights-a-week television.

We would send ever more far-fetched storylines and character notes up to the company Big Cheeses, and always the instruction would come back down again: 'Take it down market, make it sexier, more visual'. Eventually we reached a scenario for Episode One where, in the opening scene, two of the practice partners were to be having a quickie before Monday morning surgery; and later, as the credits rolled, the registrar would be giving her trainer head during a tutorial. Reality TV being then in its infancy, I baulked and quit. The programme was never made.

Andrew Bax and Radcliffe were as gracious as I was embarrassed when I hightailed it back to their offices, once more available for work. Within the year, I was writing again for the Green Journal; not about books, but under the regular headline of *Inner sense*. (*Inner* to match my previous titles; *Inner sense* as an affectionate tribute to a GP educator known for his fondness for the phrase 'in a sense'; and for its allusion to 'wide-eyed innocence'.) I was allowed to create the fictitious academic post of 'Radcliffe Armchair of Clinical Philosophy', and appoint myself the Armchair Professor, with a special interest in the emerging discipline of Contemplative Research.

Beneath this flimflam lay a measure of serious intent. I genuinely believe the privilege of being a clinician gives one powerful credentials in fields such as ethics, logic and epistemology, which are commonly the preserve of philosophers. I also believe that philosophical tenets and principles central to clinical practice can be discovered while seated in one's armchair, lost in contemplation. For two years, *Inner sense* gave me a platform for improvisations upon this theme, decorated with intellectual cadenzas which lurched erratically from the erudite to the tricksy, and brought me (not a moment too soon) face to face with my own inner smart-arse. But it was fun while it lasted.

And then, just as this particular over-bucketed well began to run dry, Alec Logan, Deputy Editor of the *British Journal of General Practice*, invited me to do a monthly column for the *Back Pages*, the *BJGP*'s comment and opinion section. This time I settled on the running title *Behind the lines*.

I'm passionate about the Royal College of GPs, the things it stands for, and its potential to add value to every aspect of primary care. I've been one of its Membership examiners for 20 years, and was Convenor of the Panel of Examiners (in effect, Chief Examiner) from 1997 to 2002. Working with the College has nourished my own career and brought me heaps of friends. But I've sometimes thought, maverick that I am, that, like all institutions, the College's systems could seem to get in the way of effectiveness. And I thought – the truest friend being an honest one – the best place to give it critical support would be from 'behind the lines'.

One of Alec's great virtues as an Editor is the way he encourages his authors to go just that little bit further than might be thought safe. The first *Behind the lines* was scheduled to appear in January 2002. So, given a four-week lead-in time, I was writing it in November 2001, shortly after the events in America of September 11th. Possibly because of the intense emotions of that time, possibly because my own mother's death was still achingly recent – whatever the reason, while writing the New York piece I was aware of a soft crescendo of purpose, like the gentle tug of a weary dog on a lead when he smells home. Like other, more eminent columnists, I found that the attempt to make, let alone to express in 800 words, connections between global outrage and our own parochial little agenda felt hideously disrespectful; yet at the same time it seemed the only respect open to me to pay.

When scared and under attack, everybody needs a champion. Patients do, and seek to make champions out of their doctors. We professionals do too, when we feel overstretched and misunderstood. At such times we cast our trade associations and Royal Colleges in the champion role. Yet because we realise that champions are created out of our own weakness, and we shouldn't really need them, we salve our ambivalence by chastising our champions for their mortal limitations.

Writing that first *Behind the lines* column, I seemed to hear, more clearly than I had before, the voice of my own private values. In hindsight, having been elected in 2003 to the Presidency of the RCGP – and I swear I had no conscious inkling of it at the time – I suspect it was a manifesto.

* * *

Knowing you have a column to write every month produces an intense but episodic kind of arousal. The Celia Johnson and Trevor Howard characters in *Brief Encounter* would know what I mean. For most of the time between deadlines life goes on, un-annotated and un-critiqued. Occasionally an idea strikes – though usually not (or such has been my experience) an idea for a Big Theme, nor even for a Topical Topic. More often what has me reaching for the little black notebook will be an Opening Sentence. 'General practice is the art of managing disappointment', for example. Or, 'The new GP contract is tough on quality, tough on the causes of quality.' One-liners like this, I find, are usually enough to start the juices flowing. And luckily, they do tend to emerge from the unconscious in the nick of time as delivery day approaches. Then, once a starter is safely down on the empty page, the solitary business of crafting a piece will generally gather pace. A good opening sentence is the literary equivalent of foreplay to the sin of Onan.

To wordsmiths like me, who profess not to know what they think until they see what they say, the obvious riposte should be, 'Well keep quiet till you *do!*' But silence is not an option for the columnist with a commitment, let alone a contract. What is compulsory (and what becomes compulsive) is the regular flow of self-examination: discovering with each fresh assignment what it is that seems to matter and what seems to be individual. The empty page is a still surface; into it is tossed the germ of an idea, and through the ripples of its impact one may dive into one's own dark waters, finding a voice and creating a persona on the way down.

Mind you, there are some pretty scary creatures down there, denizens of the psychic deeps. The author of an opinion column may set out to trawl for wit and insight, but lots of other less attractive things get dredged up and brought ashore. In my own case I am regularly confronted with my own preachiness and paranoia; my own cynicism, intolerance and pedantry; my love of showing off; my preference for the undercover sniper's position over that of leader of the cavalry charge. Of these vices, the one I am least ashamed of is cynicism. A cynic, I reckon, is just a natural coward trying to act brave. That's me. Given how much of the evidence of progress trumpeted by our policy-makers is phoney, and given how widespread is the State belief that pseudo-care is as good as the genuine article, I think there is plenty of need for bravery and plenty of excuse for cowardice.

Nevertheless, these periodic voyages into my own beliefs have reassured me about a lot of things too. I still know that being a GP is the best job in the world. I'm still convinced that the generalist way of doing medicine gives greater scope for respecting the humanity of both patient and doctor than does the specialist[5]. I believe my professional values have remained those of the consulting room, where nothing is more important than the other person sharing that privileged loneliness. I think that 'care' should be a verb, not a commodity. I know what

---

[5] David Haslam put it neatly when, introduced to another doctor at a party, he enquired, 'Are you a generalist, or just a partialist?'

fun teaching is, showing younger colleagues the tricks and delights of the trade. I support everything the Royal College of GPs stands for, and nearly everything it does. I know that all institutions, like people, are flawed. But while flaws in people are often endearing, and are to be understood and tolerated, flaws in institutions — State and professional — are not.

The present volume is a compilation mainly of articles, excerpts and columns taken from the Green Journal and the *Back Pages* of the *BJGP*, clustered around a number of recurring themes. I've selected pieces that made me chuckle, or moistened my eye, or (occasionally) made my jaw clench in a Bulldog Drummond kind of way. If further justification is called for, Jack Point in Gilbert and Sullivan's *Yeomen of the guard* will sing it for me:

> I can teach you with a quip if I've a mind,
> I can trick you into learning with a laugh;
> Oh, winnow all my folly, folly, folly and you'll find
> A grain or two of truth among the chaff.

Musing thus, I returned to that paean of the Zen experience, Sosan's song of enlightenment *On faith in the heart*, and read:

> The more talking and thinking, the more astray you go.
> Do not seek for the truth, only cease to cherish opinions.

And thus reproached, what's a self-opinionated scribbling quack to do, except mutter 'Bugger' under his breath and keep on trying?

2

Events, dear boy

So said Harold Macmillan, Prime Minister 1957–1963, when asked what his biggest problem was.

Doctors' professional problems (or at least, the problems that have us reaching for our professional hats) tend to be, as events go, rather small beer. A new GP contract, the latest recruitment and retention statistics, today's drug scare, a fresh clutch of Department of Health targets, the supplanting of the Joint Committee on Postgraduate Training for General Practice by the Postgraduate Medical Education and Training Board – none of them exactly stops the spinning world on its axis. By contrast, when some large-scale disaster or triumph occurs – famine, royal marriage or Rugby World Cup final – it is usually in our capacity as private individuals that we react.

But occasionally the magnitude of an event, or our corporate involvement in it, presses both personal and professional buttons. The attacks on New York and Washington of September 11th 2001; the death of Princess Diana in Paris, August 31st 1997; the aftermath of the murderous career of the appalling Dr Harold Shipman: all impacted on general practice as well as on individual GPs. The first piece in this section, written in November 2001, was also my first *Behind the lines* column for the *Back Pages*.

On the events of September 11th[1]

Coffee poured, I'm ready to begin what was once called 'writing'. An intimidating white screen, labelled 'New Blank Document' and destined to become my inaugural column for *Back Pages*, is mouse-clicked into existence. Inconsequential thoughts arise, tantalise, evaporate – 'In the beginning was Microsoft Word ...'

Some good advice comes to mind – 'Write about what matters to you.' OK, so what matters? Revalidation? The College's working party on cradle cap? No; since the cataclysmic events of September 11th, hardly anything has seemed to matter as much as the concatenation of atrocity that began that day in New York and Washington.

The images are seared into our collective memory – airliners coming out of a clear blue sky and bringing down the emblems of America's domination of the world's agenda. But, in every sense except the literal, the sky was anything but clear and blue. The backdrop to the outrage was black with hatred, green with dollar bills, blood-red with history.

---

[1] *Behind the lines*, Back Pages, *Brit. J. Gen. Pract.*, January 2002.

Hollywood knows that, for a movie to feel like it matters, the characters, even the bad guys, must have a back-story – a past that makes sense of their behaviour – and the Act III climax must catapult them into an unseen but all-too-imaginable future. It's drummed into every aspiring screenwriter: 'Think the big picture before you write the small one'. That is (or should be) what President Bush's friends are telling him now. We have little to send but love to those who grieve amidst the rubble of Manhattan. Instead, our contribution to the healing process should be informed with the best thoughtfulness we can muster, and that means thinking the big picture.

Some commentators on both sides of the Atlantic have found the courage to wonder why the USA – land of the free, the self-fulfilled and the self-obsessed – should find itself so violently loathed. And if there is to be any healing power in friendship, America's friends should help her dare to see a picture big enough to contain the answer. It will have to be done gently yet insistently; for any answer will come in terms of that nation's reputation as a bully and a know-all – cosmopolitan, vibrant and creative by all means, but, at least as far its conduct abroad is concerned, a bully and a know-all nevertheless.

It is, I suppose, progress that the definition of 'enemy' has been expanded beyond particular individuals. I suppose it makes a bigger picture for the war to be against an abstract noun, 'terrorism'. Yet the dead in America and Afghanistan surely deserve better than to be thought of just as ideological casualties, collateral damage in a philosophical war-game. These particular dead should not have needed to die at all. In a war between abstractions, better weapons than airliners, B-52s and smart bombs would be other abstractions – listening, humility, generosity, mutual regard, even the apparently forgotten religious virtues of compassion and forgiveness.

'Only connect ...' wrote E M Forster. I'm afraid talk of bullies and know-alls inescapably reminds me of the present British government, and indeed of *all* our recent governments. For if sabotage and subversion are the politics of the powerless, the extremities to which the unheard and the desperate are driven when their aspirations are overridden by a complacent Establishment, then maybe some of our own institutions, notably the NHS, are at risk of catastrophic attack out of a seemingly clear blue sky.

Doctors and patients alike know to their cost that the shameful inadequacy of Britain's health service has not been cured by cosmetic surgery to its management structure or by homeopathic doses of money. They also know that their protestations are systematically ignored, denied, belittled and dismissed by our bullying know-all governments.

General practice has been called the art of managing uncertainty. If only it were that simple. In the consulting room and in our wider professional lives we are having to acquire a new skill – managing disappointment and desperation, our patients' and our own. And with that new skill may have to come a new role – the GP, if not as social terrorist, as freedom fighter.

The College[2], like the NHS, is in danger of withering for lack of resources. Many young doctors who pass the MRCGP exam don't continue as fee-paying members. Why? Because they don't see the College as standing for the things that

---

[2] The Royal College of General Practitioners. Its Membership examination ('the MRCGP exam') is taken by the vast majority of GP Registrars as they come to the end of their vocational training.

really matter. And what matters supremely, I believe, is that the impoverishment of Britain's emasculated health service is, on behalf of its consumers and its providers, exposed and rammed home to Government before damagingly confrontational tactics become the only option for the disillusioned. The College has the people and organisation to lead creative protest. Has it the nerve to think the big picture?

Faking it[3]

How's best to say this? Do you perhaps remember there was a bit of a hoo-ha after some sociological pundit dared to imply that a degree of public humbug might have attended the obsequies of the late Princess of Wales? Well – and I wouldn't admit this to just anybody – on hearing this, I thought, with all due respect, 'Actually, I agree.'

I mean, personal and private tragedy I grant you. As doctors we don't need lessons from anybody in the agonies of bereavement, nor in the processes of projection that left millions ostensibly more distraught over the death of a glamorous stranger than all the unmentionable sadnesses and unfairnesses in their own lives. But, as the reports begin to come in of plaster effigies of the departed being seen to weep mascara tears, I can't have been the only one wondering what Kraken had awoken in the depths of the national psyche.

The piece that caused the stir was a chapter by Anthony O'Hear, Professor of Philosophy at Bradford, in *Faking it: the sentimentalisation of modern society*[4]. It is published by The Social Affairs Unit, which, according to *The Times*, 'is famous for driving its coach and horses through the liberal consensus, scattering intellectual picket lines as it goes, (and) for raising questions which strike people most of the time as too dangerous or difficult to think about.'

'Sentimentalisation' as defined in *Faking it* means the tendency endemic in the institutions of *fin de siècle* Britain for the private avoidance of painful truths to be compensated by an exaggerated but sham public display of concern. The sentimentalist hopes that posturing, if sufficiently flamboyant, will pass for genuine commitment. Sentimentality – some would call it hypocrisy – is the politician who in well-rounded phrases at the bedside of the cancer victim denounces smoking, yet opposes an advertising ban. It's the churchgoer ever ready to quote the parable of the good Samaritan at his quarrelsome children, yet who has never bought a copy of *The big issue* in his life. Or the scandalous myth that the damage caused by and to uncherished and undisciplined schoolchildren can be prevented by publishing league tables of the schools they truant from. Sentimentalisation is the creative force behind the pot noodle.

Faking it contains a short but superb analysis of how medicine is shot through with sentimentality. Bruce Charlton has contributed an essay on the extent to which the laity has succumbed to acclaiming the ersatz, the phoney and the unsubstantiated in medicine. The alternatives – complexity, disappointment and powerlessness in the face of nature – are simply too painful to contemplate.

---

[3] Excerpted from 'Neighbour on books', *Education for General Practice* (1998), **9**, 382–6.
[4] Anderson D and Mullen P (eds) (1998) *Faking it: the sentimentalisation of modern society*. The Social Affairs Unit, London.

Charlton attempts, persuasively on the whole, to expose as sentimental bunkum such credos of the *Guardian*-reading classes as complementary medicine, counselling and consumerism. 'People,' he writes, 'would *like* fringe medicine to be true, just as they would like *The wind in the willows* to be true.' And, 'The combination of therapeutic ineffectuality, spiritual arrogance and moral bankruptcy mark out psychotherapy as one of the great scandals of our era.'

Some of the pieces in *Faking it* are over the top: shrill, sharp, wobbly sopranos in an otherwise balanced chorus. But readers of this Journal have a good enough ear to filter out the excesses, and will, I confidently predict, delight in it.

On Shipmania[5]

Harold Shipman's come and gone, like a rent boy. At least you'd think so, reading the newspapers. 304 column inches in *The Times* the week of Dame Janet Smith's report[6], and since then – nothing. Mind you, I'm sure those hundreds of families lacerated with grief, doubt and recrimination haven't been able to draw so neat a line under his wickedness, nor to move on in quite so slick a fashion. And neither have we, for GPs too have been indirectly hurt in the fall-out.

Much of the press initially seemed to concur with the BMA's[7] assessment that the Shipman affair was a 'tragic systems error', requiring some urgent and important (but not conceptually difficult) procedural reforms. The instinctive response, said the *Independent on Sunday*, was 'to express horror at the unique brutality, and move on.' 'His psychopathic behaviour,' said the editorial writer of the *Daily Mirror*, 'should not affect our attitude to the medical profession.'

So far, so sensible. But, like compulsive hand-washers or pavement crack-avoiders, the ladies and gentlemen of the fourth estate couldn't resist the chance of a free ride on some of their favourite hobby horses. In a frenzy of non sequiturs and knight's moves that, voiced by a private citizen, would have had the Approved Social Worker knocking on the door before you could say 'Largactil', the muddled thinking began in earnest.

'It would be absurd to think a mass murderer lurked inside every doctor,' the *Daily Mirror* conceded. But the *Daily Express* snarled, 'It is time doctors admitted their own kind were as capable of wrong-doing as the rest of us and put an end to their culture of complicity and cover-up.' Complicity in – covering up – an almost unimaginable killing spree? Ouch!

The *Independent on Sunday* thought it could see the wider lesson: 'We must stop trusting our doctors so much.' So did *The Times*: 'It is vital the government does its best to ensure that the bond of trust between doctor and patient is not lost.' Well make your minds up. But either way, God help us if preserving that trust depends on a Government whose reliance on spin and silly targets has done more to undermine it than Harold Shipman ever will. I'd have thought it was our job – the profession's job – to earn and deserve patients' confidence, and government's job

---

[5] *Behind the lines*, Back Pages, *Brit. J. Gen. Pract.*, October 2002.

[6] Dame Janet Smith, a High Court judge, chaired the public inquiry into the activities of the mass murderer GP Dr Harold Shipman, and into the performance of the various statutory bodies, authorities, organisations and individuals responsible for protecting patients. The first of her five reports, *Death disguised*, was published on 19th July 2002.

[7] The British Medical Association.

to remove the impediments to it. The *Glasgow Herald* reckoned 'the real reason Shipman got away with it was that he was a popular GP,' and 'those responsible for policing doctors' had to make sure there was never another one like him. I see: doctors scoring above average on patient satisfaction questionnaires get a dawn visit from the GMC Special Branch[8]. The *Express* was sure the death toll would have been lower had Shipman been struck off when he was caught forging pethidine prescriptions in the 1970s. Or, for that matter, if the driving test examiner had failed him for clipping the kerb while reversing round a corner.

The outbreak of sophistry even penetrated Princes Gate[9]. The College was invited to submit evidence to the Smith Inquiry. At the time, I was Convenor of the MRCGP exam: and someone within the College who should have known better asked me to document the evidence that anyone who passed the examination was not a criminal psychopath. Now that's a tricky one, another example of thinking an academic tool can also be a vehicle for political posturing. To the best of my knowledge no candidate has submitted videotape of a criminal assault as part of a consulting skills assessment. The simulated surgery can't really afford to sacrifice any of its role-players. And in my experience candidates in the orals, asked whether they are homicidal maniacs, tend to say 'No.' So I told the someone-who-should-have-known-better that the exam did not, and had no plans to, include a Serial Killer Identification Module. We could, I suggested, ask exam applicants for a testimonial signed by a Chief Constable and forensic psychiatrist. But for all I know, examined on his care of those patients he forbore to slay, Dr Shipman could quite possibly have done rather well in the MRCGP.

GPs can stand the funny remarks when, post-Shipman, we draw up the Depo-Provera or manipulate a torticollis. But when we find ourselves caught up in generic slanging that implies we're collectively untrustworthy, or accessories to slaughter, or inappropriately qualified, or dangerous in proportion to our popularity, we too have become victims – not of a lone assassin but of damaging category errors. They need to be soundly refuted, and ourselves vociferously defended, by the professional bodies to whom we pay subscriptions.

---

[8] The General Medical Council; the statutory body charged with regulating doctors' fitness to practise.
[9] 14 Princes Gate, London; headquarters of the Royal College of General Practitioners.

3

. . . with a small 'p'

I agree with the late Will Rogers[1]: 'The more you read and observe about this Politics thing, you got to admit that each party is worse than the other.' I doubt I am alone in believing it was Margaret Thatcher and Kenneth Clarke who pulled the plug on decency in the NHS when, with fund-holding, they introduced a competitive internal market into general practice. Nor am I alone, I suspect, in being disappointed that the Blair government seems to have no remedy but to insist a square plug will seal the leak.

Part of the trouble, as the piece *On heroes* suggests, is the five-year parliamentary cycle, with its inevitable imperative that everything has to be made to look successful in time for the next election. The corollary is the Law of Quinquennial Paralysis: 'In year n of a five-year Parliament, no policy dare be adopted which requires more than $(5 - n)$ years to appear effective.' The folly of this situation, and the impotence of 'big picture thinking' in the face of political expediency, is pointed up in *On quality and quantity*, specifically in relation to the GP recruitment issue.

Two pieces in this chapter address recent changes to GPs' working arrangements. *On tents*, written shortly before compulsory GP appraisals were introduced in April 2003, reflects my ambivalence about the educational versus the regulatory objects of the exercise, an ambivalence which is still unresolved even as this book goes to press.

In August 2002, when *On contracts and panopticons* appeared, our negotiators were recommending the profession adopt the new contract which had been recently proposed, under which GPs could buy out of many of what had hitherto been core responsibilities, and could be richly rewarded for working obediently to a large array of performance targets. I suspected the new contract would be a bit like the electronic tags worn by prisoners in the community, which alert the authorities if the offender strays away from the officially approved home range. In the event, GPs voted to approve the new contract by a majority of four to one, and it was implemented in April 2004. As to whether the greater earning potential will prove hard bought in terms of lost freedom and respect, time will tell.

The remaining pieces are commentaries on two books, each offering striking or satirical analogies for the political process. The first is a reworking of a Confucian manual on the art of war. The other is a vitriolic but hilarious denunciation of the pettiness of politics as practised in the University of Cambridge a century ago, *Microcosmographia academica* by F M Cornforth. My friend David Haslam used

---

[1] Will Rogers (1879–1935). American vaudeville entertainer and master of the political one-liner, e.g. 'Every time Congress makes a joke it's law, and every time they make a law it's a joke.'

also to write a regular column for the Green Journal, *Haslam on Education*. For one issue we swopped; he did books and I did education. I devoted my 'education' column chiefly to the *Microcosmographia*, and — so much had I enjoyed it — reviewed it shortly afterwards in the 'books' pages. Both articles are reprinted here.

On heroes[2]

One of the weekend papers has a regular column where a C-list celebrity is asked a formulaic series of personal questions, and answers them in terms calculated to give the illusion of frankness. 'What's your greatest fear?' 'Which living person apart from Margaret Thatcher do you most despise?' That sort of thing. I confess — but I bet you do it too — sometimes it's fun to imagine one's own replies, witty and evasive for the most part, but with occasional glimpses of the lovable sage we all know we are at heart. 'How often do you have sex?' (When I remember.) 'Do you believe in life after death?' (I'll get back to you on that.)

There's always one question I have no difficulty with: 'Which historical figure do you most admire?' Easy, no doubt about it — Schubert. To me, the composer Franz Schubert is the patron saint of the little guy. Small in stature, colossal in creative legacy, loyal to and cherished by his many intimate friends, Schubert could be alone in the midst of a crowd, his imagination constantly translating the human predicament in all its poignancy into musical form. Someone wrote, '... whereas with Mozart at his best we scale the heights and come down again, when Schubert is at his best we can plumb the soul's absolute depths and come up again.'[3] What a great doctor Schubert would have made; yet arguably how impoverished would have been posterity had he devoted himself to the merely corporeal instead of the sublime.

Heroes have the ability to induce improvement at a distance, to enrich (often unwittingly) admirers remote in time and place, to teach without teaching. Heroism is out of fashion nowadays, when everything may be put into league tables except the things that matter. But I think it's OK to have heroes, as long as the hero has merit as well as talent. Ah, but how are we to determine merit, especially if the hero-designate is long dead? Legions of could-have-been should-have-been heroes have passed unacknowledged into history, solely because we fail to spot the equivalences between their times and ours, between the adversities they transcended and those we wrongly believe to be uniquely our own.

Let me now make the case for dumpy myopic little Schubert. That his talent was prodigious we'll take as read. But merit? You'd think that — middle class, secure, miffed but not devastated at the modesty of his reputation — Schubert experienced little adversity against which to test his potential as a hero. (Except the syphilis that killed him at 31, of course, which frankly he didn't handle well; fancy swallowing all that mercury without checking the side-effects.)

When Schubert began writing songs in the early 1800s, they were expected to conform to a 'strophic' structure: each verse written to pretty much the same music, each verse closing with a pretty cadence. Hardly surprising: Schubert's

[2] *Behind the lines*, Back Pages, *Brit. J. Gen. Pract.*, April 2003.
[3] Actually it was me. The paper from which this quotation is taken is reprinted as Chapter 12 of this book.

Vienna was itself a conformist and rigidly structured city. But, behind its chocolate box façade, Vienna was in fact a police state, permeated by spies and corruption, presided over by the Blairite Prince Metternich and his henchman, the Alistair Campbell-like Chief of Police, Josef Sedlnitzky. Schubert's friend Bauernfeld wrote of a regime that 'weighed on us all like a monkey we could not get off our back'. Martha Wilmot complained that 'we never cough nor wipe a child's nose without the event being reported to Government'. Individuality was dangerous. Safety lay in a public show of smiling acquiescence, following the guidelines, staying (as we should now say) 'on message'.

Encouraged perhaps by braver friends, Schubert made a small but crucial change to musical convention. He began to write some songs *durchkomponiert* – 'through-composed'. Rather than being compartmentalised into repetitious verses, the text was set to a single over-arching and coherent plan, freely but faithfully following the logic and mood of the words. The big picture became more important than its component parts. By his own lights, Schubert's innovation was subversive, seditious – but (as the triumph of imagination over regulation) oh! how liberating.

My point? Our national life and institutions are strophically constrained to the tune of our five-year electoral cycle. Every five years the NHS has to be made to look neat, to sound pretty, to act obedient. Government, for fear of short-term unpopularity, dares not think the big picture that the complexity of healthcare requires. So – since we are middle class, secure and miffed at the modesty of our reputation – we must encourage it. Social policy needs to be more *durchkomponiert*. Sorry about the ugliness of the phrase, but Schubert can teach us anti-compartmentalism. And for that he is a hero.

On quality and quantity[4]

There is no single issue more important to the improved health of the nation than the drive for quality, to whose mast the RCGP has firmly Blu-tacked its colours. Top quality clinical medicine is – or should be – within the intellectual reach of every doctor. And a steady narrowing of the gap between aspiration and reality is – or should be – the experience of every voting tax-paying patient. We know pretty much how it is to be done. Non-threatening incentives to promulgate best practice. A ratcheting-up of the present 'minimal competence' level of summative assessment. Replacing the culture of blame with a culture of cooperation and common sense. Vocational training based in general practice. And so on. Investment; time; resources. The long haul; the big picture; the non-partisan vision. Pursue the drive for quality, and the nation's blood pressure will soon be impeccable, its cholesterol level beyond reproach. Patients in their droves will scarcely have time to scribble a 'thank you' note to their GPs before they're up on the operating table having their veins done.

On the other hand, there is no single issue more important to the improved health of the nation than the drive for quantity, to whose mast the Department of Health has firmly nailed its colours. Nailed? Would it were anything so flimsy. Riveted, welded, superglued. The logic is at first sight irresistible – more care for patients requires more appointments and more time, and hence more doctors.

More doctors means more recruits, faster training, fewer failures, fewer drop-outs. But since we apparently need about another 6000 GPs by a week on Tuesday, they are not going to be delivered by what we've come to regard as the normal channels.

So the chicanery has already started. The press gangs have set to work recruiting GPs from Spain and Austria, wooing them with fables of that healthcare paradise which is the UK. The (so far) very few who have been seduced will have their expectations quickly down-sized to British levels and will be fast-tracked into practice in the most disadvantaged areas. Deaneries are already under pressure from the DoH to lower their selection and training standards, and one at least has been told that the answer 'no' is unacceptable. The embryonic Postgraduate Medical Education and Training Board (from whose title the word 'Standards' has interestingly been quietly dropped) will have most of its 25 members appointed by the Secretary of State, to whom alone it will be accountable.

For some reason I find myself remembering a little scene I saw being played out at my local garden centre this morning. Judging by the scrum around the wallflowers, you'd think they were giving away a crate of Beaujolais nouveau with every half-box. The adults were tight-lipped and ruthless, elbows flying, trolleys cutting swathes through the competition like the war chariots of Boadicea. But the under-fives were having a whale of a time. The centre has rather a nice take on the shopping trolley; some of them, for the use of parents with imaginative children, are got up as toy cars. While the grown-up pushes towards whatever it is the grown-up wants, Junior is seated behind a red plastic steering wheel. The wheel, of course, is connected to nothing at all. Nevertheless, 'Brrmm brrrmmm!' goes the kiddy, engrossed in a private fantasy of power and control, steering vigorously to the left in the direction of the preserves and biscuits. And the other shoppers smile indulgently. But today the wallflowers were over there, to the right.

Quality and quantity agendas, as currently formulated, are irreconcilable. 'Better equals fewer' and 'more equals worse' are simultaneous equations with no solution. Unless – brainwave! – the College, which continues to cherish the hope that MRCGP will become the entrance standard to unsupervised practice, can increase the exam's pass rate to 185%. That should do it. But otherwise the College's policy of 'promoting excellence in family medicine' may make us the enemies of the Department, whose imperative is to do a quick paint job on the NHS in time for the next election. Diplomacy, persuasiveness, and an unblinking gaze are required of our leaders, and we should pray for them now as never before. In the short to medium term, our quality agenda puts us potentially in the same relationship to Government as a hedgehog to a truck.

We can console ourselves that hedgehogs, as a species, multiply and survive, while trucks ultimately turn to rust. Meanwhile though, it would be sad if the last that was heard of us for a bit was a happy 'Brrmm brrrmmm!' dying away on the indifferent air.

On tents[5]

The week between Christmas and New Year is an odd time. The shift from disgraceful self-indulgence to Puritan resolution will sometimes cause a spiritual

---

[5] *Behind the lines*, Back Pages, Brit. J. Gen. Pract., February 2003.

abyss to open up, a kind of long dark spastic colon of the soul. Into this void may come visions; but whether they be profundities or merely the products of fermentation is for someone else to judge. Anyway: as I nibbled one last *marron glacé* before breaking in the new running shoes I thought now's as good a time as any to fill in my annual – my first – GP appraisal form. (Now come on, of *course* you've heard of appraisal.) And lo! as I did attempt to answer question 3 on page 2 of Form 3 ('*What professional or personal factors significantly constrain you in maintaining and developing your skills and knowledge?*') I fell into a dream. And in my dream I was carried unto an high place, whence I saw spread before me even like unto a tented village. And behold! the name of the tented village was General Practice.

Tents, as we know, are of two kinds, classified according to the *locus micturendi*. There are those – let us call them type A – where the golden stream is directed outwards from within. And there is type B. Most of us (if the image is not too unpleasant) have a foot in each, but a predilection for only one. I tend to be a type B man myself. Cynic that I am, I'm usually more alert to the muddle and palm-greasing that spawn the latest good idea than I am to the lofty principles its advocates claim for it. Show me a PCO[6] or a clinical protocol or a new contract, and I'll show you a wigwam whereinto my instincts are to point Percy, as it were, *ab exteriore*.

But with appraisal it's been different. Appraisal, when first mooted, struck me as a tent it might be better to be on the inside of. I am, after all, passionately convinced that guided introspection is the best driver of adult learning. And if state-controlled and contractually-required appraisals are the closest we can come, in this near-totalitarian NHS, to genuinely formative reflection – well, I thought, I'll try and make it work. So I put my hand up as a potential appraiser, and in due course (having signed an affidavit to the effect that I was not, as far as I knew, the subject of an ongoing criminal investigation) was approved. I am now licensed, as Sir Liam Donaldson[7] has so memorably expressed it, to help my local colleagues 'consolidate and improve on good performance aiming towards excellence in a positive and supportive developmental process'. Gulp. It is *not* the primary business of an appraiser to denounce a duff doc, merely to help him or her to burst into tears and promise to try harder. We remain, after all, a caring profession.

We appraisers thought it best to apply the Delphic injunction, 'Appraise thyself'. So, in order to get a bit of practice and street cred under our belts, we're all doing each other before we go live. X is doing Y, who's doing Z, who's doing X; no chance, you see, of my overlooking your shortcomings if you'll overlook mine.

But here's an interesting question, slipped unobtrusively into Form 3, page 6: '*What safeguards are in place to ensure propriety in your . . . use of your professional position?*' In other words, are you Harold Shipman? No I'm bloody not. And if I were, what would I put? 'Curses, you got me bang to rights, I'm a murdering psychopath'? It would be interesting to ask him. 'Dear Harold, I enclose Form 3, to be returned in complete confidence ahead of our forthcoming appraisal meeting.'[8]

---

[6] Primary Care Organisation: the local conglomerate responsible for purchasing secondary care and other services on behalf of GPs. Slightly more cooperative than the fund-holding practices of the 1980s, but similarly motivated.

[7] The Chief Medical Officer.

[8] Harold Shipman committed suicide in prison, January 12th 2004.

Oh dear; it's so hard to stay starry-eyed. Maybe I have to redefine appraisal as a type B tent after all, a token exercise in anti-Shipmanism best watered from outside. But there are so many tents, a whole village of them. Clinical governance. Revalidation. Summative assessment. MRCGP. National Service Frameworks. The new contract. So many issues where whether you are inside or outside the tent is arbitrary, irrational and ultimately inconsequential, but which, to the individual, seem to matter enormously.

There are two things about tented villages. The first is that they are congregations of the dispossessed, places of hunger, impoverishment and squalor, places where fights are always breaking out, temporary encampments that need urgently to be replaced with more dignified and worthy structures. Secondly, tented villages are the backdrop for countless unsung cameos of individual heroism, self-sacrifice, nobility. Tented villages are where *médecins sans frontières* come into their own. If it's not an insult to these intrepid guys, maybe in a small way we too could aspire to be GPs *sans frontières*, the takers-down of tents in our own vernacular wilderness.

On contracts and panopticons[9]

I love a nice metaphor, don't you? The 'Caritas' rose, for example, specially developed and named to mark 50 years of the College's presence on the block. *Cum scientia caritas*:[10] 'where there is science, let flowers bloom' – how very sixties. Be that as it may, I bought two of them. They are now flourishing in tubs on either side of the steps leading down from the decking where, Pimms in hand, I sprawl of a warm summer eve planning a little light gardening tomorrow. And the metaphor? The College rose, I discover, has a lovely scent but drops its petals in the slightest wind.

Equally deserving of being shoved outside in the rain and liberally sprinkled with manure is the new draft contract, whose potential to transform the fortunes of general practice our negotiators have invited us to endorse in the first part of a two-stage referendum. Stage one: 'Is it a basis for detailed financial discussion?' Stage two: 'Finance being agreed, shall we go for it?' I and every colleague I've spoken to have been agonising over whether it's best to give the proposals the thumbs down right from the start, in order not to waste anybody's time, or leave the *nolle prosequi* until later, on the grounds that at least the powers that be can't then say we never even considered them.

June Council[11] debated the proposals, which was good of it, given how little effective input the College has had into them. Council on these occasions always puts me in mind of the old *Punch* cartoon showing father and son on the beach, the former posed heroically at the breakers' edge. 'Roll on, thou mighty ocean, roll!', he apostrophises; and the boy gazes up at him admiringly, saying, 'Oh look, daddy, it's doing it.'

---

[9] *Behind the lines*, Back Pages, *Brit. J. Gen. Pract.*, August 2002.
[10] *Cum scientia caritas*: the motto of the Royal College of General Practitioners, it means 'combining knowledge with compassion'.
[11] The governing and trustee body of the Royal College of General Practitioners.

Members seemed all set to salute the new contract, early speakers 'Good show'-ing and 'Just the ticket'-ing in appreciative chorus. Then one of my favourite ladies, Iona Heath (whom I once delighted by nicknaming 'Tinkerbell', after the irascible fairy in *Peter Pan*[12]), sprang to her incisive feet. If concrete-sounding things like outcome frameworks, quality ladders, controlled workloads and money were to be dumped on us, she suggested (and I paraphrase), general practice would in consequence suffer a debilitating loss of abstract nouns, such as freedom, humanity and – her own particular favourite – mystery. Attagirl. In the stiffening breeze of Iona's rhetoric, Council shed a few petals and adjourned to the kitchen to cook up some fudge.

All of which brings me naturally to Jeremy Bentham (1748–1832), English philosopher, economist and theoretical jurist, and to his best-known scheme – a design for a model prison called the 'Panopticon'.

Picture, if you will, a ring of individual cells each containing a single prisoner. The cells are well lit, having a large window in their outer wall and an even larger one facing inwards. The walls between adjacent cells are, however, solid; no inmate may catch sight of any other. At the centre of the ring is a control tower containing the guards, with blinds so arranged that, although every cell is at all times completely visible from the tower, the guards them-selves cannot be seen. The prisoner in the Panopticon never knows from one moment to the next whether or not he is being watched. Indeed, the tower may often actually be empty. But the belief that he is under constant and omniscient scrutiny leads the inmate, in effect, to police himself. Isolated from his fellows, unable to organise or collaborate, and under conditions of con-stant visibility, real or imagined, his undesirable behaviour would wither and his errant spirit be tamed. The Panopticon, Bentham crowed, was 'a new mode of obtaining power of mind over mind, in a quantity hitherto without example'; its effects would be 'morals reformed, health preserved, industry invigorated, instruction diffused'.

Although the Panopticon was never built, we can be sure it would in fact have resulted in atrophy, not ennoblement, of the spirit – mindless compliance with the regime's expectations. Sullen acquiescence is not the same as endorsement freely and joyfully given.

Remember this when you read our proposed new contract, especially the bits where it says that a light touch of central control will 'revitalise general practice and rekindle GPs' enthusiasm', while being 'based on high trust, low bureaucracy principles'.

Although Bentham conceived his Panopticon for the corrective discipline of criminals, the principle of 'the unseen overseer' can, as Michel Foucault points out, be applied wherever many are to be controlled by few[13]. Where recalcitrant children are to be controlled by teachers, for example. Or disruptive demon-strators by police, or inefficient workers by time and motion consultants.

Or independent general practice by the Department of Health. I love a nice metaphor, don't you?

---

[12] *See* Chapter 9, page 86.
[13] Foucault M, trans. Sheridan A (1991) *Discipline and punish: the birth of the prison.* Penguin Books, Harmondsworth.

The art of war for executives[14]

If you want something practical, specific and up to date by way of guidance on how to keep one step ahead of the rest, you need the philosophical generalities from 25 centuries ago of Sun Tzu's classic brought up to date by Donald Krause, *The art of war for executives*[15].

Sun Tzu was a contemporary of Confucius, and the very devil at military strategy. His teachings on warfare translate superbly and unashamedly into many a modern context, for he recognised that success is based on effective leadership. Battles are won by the organisation or person who has the greatest competitive advantage and who makes the fewest mistakes. The ideal general wins the war before the fighting begins, by developing his character over time and by positioning himself advantageously. Sun Tzu's army, like most effective organisations, has three characteristics. It exists for a defined purpose. It is information-based. And it is flexible and adaptable. Ten principles:

* learn to fight, i.e. set store by being competitive
* show the way, i.e. lead from the front
* do it right, i.e. make your actions effective
* know the facts; manage your sources and channels of information
* expect the worst; make preparations against set-backs
* seize the day, i.e. grab a quick victory when you can
* burn the bridges, i.e. make defeat intolerable
* do it better; innovate and surprise
* pull together, through organisation and training
* keep them guessing; 'What does it matter if a competitor has greater resources? If I control the situation, he cannot use them'.

If ever you needed convincing that expository prose is vastly inferior to metaphor as a vehicle for motivation and insight, this book will do it. Late of an evening, when it's time to set thought aside and just let your dreams resonate, the spirit of Sun Tzu could inspire you. 'There are five character flaws which are dangerous for a general. If he is reckless, his men can be killed. If he is cowardly, his army can be captured. If he is short-tempered, he will react in anger. If he is self-important, he can be deceived. If he is attached to his men, he will hesitate at a crucial moment. These five flaws are certainly unfortunate for the general, but they cause great destruction in war. They cause generals to fail and armies to die. Consider them well.'

Sun Tzu would have made a good GP. But an even better Secretary of State for Health.

University politics 1[16]

Funny the things you come across, the odd things that some corner of your mind knows, just knows, will go nicely with the furniture in the front parlour of your

---

[14] Excerpted from 'Neighbour on books', *Education for General Practice* (1997), **8**, 273–4.
[15] Krause D (1996) *Sun Tzu: the art of war for executives*. Nicholas Brealey Publishing, London.
[16] Excerpted from 'Neighbour on education', *Education for General Practice* (1997), **8**, 369–72.

everyday life. Vocational training, summative assessment, the 'minimal' versus 'optimal' competence debate – that sort of furniture. Let me tell you about two such things I've stumbled across in the last week.

In a book called *Hare brain, tortoise mind: why intelligence increases when you think less*[17] I learned that seldom far from the lips of the average Polish peasant is the adage 'Sleep faster; we need the pillows'. Some things are just not to be rushed. You can turn up the gas if the roast potatoes aren't done. But not with meringues. And I, and probably you, can recall a few GP registrars who were more of the meringue persuasion than of the roast potato, and who could have done with more than the recipe book's prescribed year in the oven[18]. After 12 months they were still soggy in the middle; to pass the 'crispness test' they needed not hotter, not more impatient pokes with an assessment package – just a bit longer. We have to get those set in authority over us to understand that.

The other thing was a matter of history, never my first love at school. At the age of seven I was taught the Scottish version of British history, in which (if memory serves) the Jameses were generally good things and the Georges bad. Then, aged nine, I upped sticks to a school in England, where the reverse was the case. Or possibly vice versa.

Anyway: I'd been a participant in the 8th Cambridge Conference on medical education. Theme of the week – standard-setting in assessment procedures. All the great and the good of the assessment world were there, your David Newbles, Geoff Normans, Sue Cases, Dave Swansons. We spent many happy hours devising new ways to prevent the young from getting away with murder, and extinguishing the last embers of leniency in the hearts of test-setters. On the last day, the conference organiser Richard Wakeford presented us all with a copy of *University politics*[19]. This is an account of academic life in Cambridge around the turn of the 20th century, and it includes F M Cornford's satirical advice to the young academic politician, *Microcosmographia academica*. And, though you might not think so, it is *a treasure*! Ponder this, and enjoy the sense of déjà vu.

In the Cambridge of 1903 the issue of the day was whether the teaching of Classics in the University, and the assessment of the knowledge of Greek in particular, stood in need of reform. A grasp of Greek vocabulary and grammar was all very well, some dons averred, but what of the *ideas* of ancient Greece? What of the wisdom and the philosophy expounded in the tracts that undergraduates were asked to translate so assiduously into prose and upon whose syntax alone they were examined in the Tripos?

Francis McDonald Cornford, a young Fellow of Trinity College, addressed the Classical Society. 'Let us recognise', he enjoined them, 'that a thorough grasp of ideas is a thing of worth, and quite distinct from a superficial "viewiness". To retain the full bulk of the old linguistic examination is precisely to encourage a hasty treatment of the new subjects. If these last are to be of real value for education, room must be cleared, and time allowed, for thoroughness in this department also.'

---

[17] Claxton G (1997) *Hare brain, tortoise mind: why intelligence increases when you think less*. Fourth Estate, London.

[18] Of the three-year prescribed period of vocational training for general practice, registrars usually spend only 12 months in general practice, and the remainder in hospital jobs.

[19] Johnson G (1994) *University politics*. Cambridge University Press, Cambridge.

UHB TRUST LIBRARY QEHB

'The truth is,' Cornford continued, 'that our most backward students produce week after week pages of stuff, of which you can hardly say more than that the words are Greek or Latin words. We stare impotently at the versions ...' (He might have been speaking of a good many of what pass in summative assessment for Registrar projects[20].)

... 'We stare impotently at the versions. Not a sentence, not a phrase, is Greek or Latin; and you can no more explain why they are not than you can explain to a deaf man why a casual series of notes is not music.' After all, 'L'essential, en effet, dans l'éducation, ce n'est pas la doctrine enseignée, c'est l'éveil'. The main thing in education is not curriculum, but insight.

Others went further than Cornford. The then Chancellor of the University considered the insistence on potential undergraduates' competence in both Greek and Latin to be politically unwise and socially undesirable. A 'Syndicate' or working party was established to consider what changes, if any, were desirable in the examinations. Eventually the Syndicate recommended that the Previous Examination (a kind of minimal competence pre-entry exam for aspiring undergraduates) should continue to assess the student's knowledge of two languages, one at least to be classical, but the other, optionally, modern.

Uproar. The Regius Professor of Greek, apoplectic, reminded the University Senate that Greek (though it might have been the Registrar audit project[21]) was 'an incomparable instrument of linguistic and literary training. The Greek mind has been the great originating mind of Europe; fertile in ideas which are still fruitful in every field of knowledge, ideas which at the Renaissance exercised a powerful influence on the transition from the medieval to the modern world. No language, no literature, is at once so ancient and so intensely modern as the Greek'.

The reaction itself provoked counter-reaction. The Downing Professor of the Laws of England confessed that, despite good teachers, he had never quite got the hang of Greek. 'But one thing he did learn, namely, to hate Greek and its alphabet, and its accents, and its accidence, and its syntax, and its prosody, and all its appurtenances; to long for the day when he would be allowed to learn something else; to vow that if he ever got rid of that thing never, never again would he open a Greek book or write a Greek word.'

Compromise loomed. The President of Queens' 'was persuaded that the true conservative course was to recognise in time the working of educational forces, which the Syndicate might perhaps be allowed to regret, but which it did not lie within their power to control, and to maintain and to forward a policy of sober and moderate reform'. The Provost of King's, albeit a lifelong Greek scholar, accepted that 'the study of Greek was right, but only for the right people. For the right people, it was the very best instrument; for the wrong people, it was the very worst'.

The Syndicate in 1905 held to its proposal that only one classical language (without specifying which) should be required in the Previous Examination. They were defeated in the vote, however, by the bussing-in of non-resident clergymen,

---

[20] GP registrars in vocational training are firmly encouraged to undertake a project or an audit of a clinical topic, in order (supposedly) to appreciate the value of research and audit.
[21] Lough JRM and Murray TS (1997) Training for audit: lessons still to be learned. *Brit. J. Gen. Pract.*, **47**, 290–2.

but for whose meddling the project — sorry, Greek — might thereupon have been unceremoniously dethroned as a *sine qua non*. Inevitably other matters, namely the establishment of an Economics Tripos, soon supplanted 'the Greek question' as the issue of the day. The letters page of the *Cambridge Review* of 9th November carried the wistful comment that 'causes which are fought with beating of drums and sending the fiery cross round the country are seldom really important, and never beneficial. What is wanted is steady reform brought about by wise legislation.'

They should cocoa! The move to establish Economics as a worthy discipline was attended by the self-same academic in-fighting. Vested interests trotted out the standard arguments against innovation. One supporter of the new Tripos was astonished at the ingenuity of members of the Senate in discovering reasons for not doing anything, and in an article in the *Cambridge Review* of May 1903 he listed 30 arguments of the 'over my dead body' mentality, including:

1   That the proposal is a new one.
2   That it is therefore a bad one.
3   That it is asked for by people outside.
4   That it is not asked for by people outside.
5   That if it were, that would be all the more reason why they should not have it.
16 That the University cannot afford it.
17 That it would be very dangerous to do anything that might tend to attract funds to the University.
20 That so-and-so is a genius, and his opinions must therefore be worthless.
21 That such-and-such is *not* a genius, and his opinions must therefore be worthless.
22 That there ought to be a comma after the word . . . in Regulation . . . line . . .
23 That Economics ought to be spelt with a small 'e'.
24 That people are more interested in their souls than in their stomachs.
25 That if they aren't they ought to be.
6   That the members of the Syndicate are amiable and well-meaning people.
30 That anyhow we aren't going to be bullied by any Syndicate. That we intend to vote against this, and any other scheme that might be brought forward. But that no one is more anxious than we are that the study of Economics should be developed in the University. And that altogether it's a great pity.

F M Cornford, a century ahead of our time, threw up his hands in despair at the parochial petty-mindedness that beset the process of 'steady reform brought about by wise legislation'. 'Are you not aware', he asked the ambitious academic politician, 'that conviction has never yet been produced by an appeal to reason, which only makes people uncomfortable? If you want to move them, you must address your arguments to prejudice and to the political motive.' Nevertheless, he continued, 'I like you the better for your illusions; but it cannot be denied that they prevent you from being effective, and if you do not become effective before you cease to want anything to be done — why, what will be the good of you?'

Plus ça change. Dream on, as you will, in your committee rooms and your ivory towers and your groves of academe. But sleep faster, because we need the pillows.

University politics 2[22]

In a previous essay, I lamented the similarities between committee warfare as practised now and in Cambridge University a century ago. Unashamedly I return to *University politics*, which is mainly reportage of interdepartmental squabbling between syllabus-setters but which contains the most witty and withering 20-page satire on what goes on in the corridors of power, F M Cornford's *Microcosmographia academica*. I need do no more than offer you delicious amuse-geule quotations from this the young academic politician's vademecum ...

'There was a time towards the end of 1914 when many people imagined that after the war human nature would be different, even better in some ways. But my friends tell me that academic human nature, at any rate, remains true to the ancient type. Moreover a short and inglorious career in a Government department has convinced me that the academic species is only one member of a genus wider than I had supposed.

'Propaganda ... defined as that branch of the art of lying which consists in very nearly deceiving your friends without quite deceiving your enemies.

'Among the parties in academic politics are the Adullamites, who are dangerous. They say to one another, "If you will scratch my back, I will scratch yours; and if you won't, I will scratch your face." That is why they succeed in getting all the money there is going.

'Nothing is ever done until every one is convinced that it ought to be done, and has been convinced for so long that it is now time to do something else. Twenty independent persons, each of whom has a different reason for not doing a certain thing, and not one of whom will compromise with any other, constitute a most effective check on the rashness of individuals.

'There is only one argument for doing something; the rest are arguments for doing nothing. The Principle of the Wedge is that you should not act justly now for fear of raising expectations that you will act still more justly in the future – expectations which you are afraid you will not have the courage to satisfy. Every public action which is not customary either is wrong, or, if it is right, is a dangerous precedent. It follows that nothing should ever be done for the first time.

'A few bad reasons for doing something neutralise all the good reasons for doing it. "I was in favour of the proposal until I hear Dr—'s arguments in support of it." '

And so blissfully on. Another of Cornford's characters is the Young Man in a Hurry. He is 'a narrow-minded and youthful prig, inexperienced enough to imagine that something might be done before very long, and even to suggest definite things. He may be known by his propensity to organise societies for the purpose of making silk purses out of sows' ears, and is afflicted with a conscience which is apt to break out, like the measles, in patches.'

Ouch. That's me off to a T.

---

[22] Excerpted from 'Neighbour on books', *Education for General Practice* (1997), **9**, 106–7.

4

The road from nowhere to nothing

Philosophy, n. A route of many roads leading from nowhere to nothing.
Ambrose Bierce, *The Devil's Dictionary*[1]

To be a doctor, and especially a GP, is to be regularly plunged into that maelstrom of misery and joy known rather loftily as 'the human condition'. Indeed, the better we become at empathising with our patients, the more drenchings we get. Scarcely a surgery goes by without our being confronted with some situation of a kind that, over the centuries, has provoked the deepest of deep thought. The mystery of life, and its debatable sanctity. The other mystery of death, and our behaviour in the face of it. The meaning of suffering; and whether to look for any meaning is itself meaningful. The suspicion some actions are right and others wrong, while others may be simply expedient or ill-advised. And underpinning everything, the unfolding drama of what it is to be a human being in relationship with other human beings.

The fact that the accomplishments of modern medicine allow us to do much *more* about these profundities than sit around and philosophise does not, I believe, justify our doing anything *less*. Anything less than sit around and philosophise, that is. It behoves us not merely to get off our butts and do something, but to sit there and think about it as well. In this chapter, I try to make a half-serious case that the medical profession has a real contribution to make to metaphysics.

The first three pieces – the 'Radcliffe armchair lectures on clinical philosophy' – were written in 1999, a time when the world of medical education was having one of its regular spells of bickering. The issue of the day was how young GPs at the end of their vocational training were to have their consultation skills assessed. Legislation requires that these doctors demonstrate that they can manage the communication side of the doctor–patient encounter, but more than one method of assessment was (and still is) in use. Unfortunately the proponents of the various methods had got themselves into a bout of arm-wrestling which dragged on for months and years until an accommodation was reached. How nice (I thought at the time, and still do) it would be if people in conflict could cut out the war and move straight to the armistice. The analysis developed in the 'Radcliffe lectures' is an attempt to work out why we find this so hard. The

---

[1] Ambrose Bierce (1842–1914). American newspaperman and satirist. *The Devil's Dictionary* (Oxford University Press, 1998 with an introduction by Roy Morris) was originally published in 1906 as *The Cynic's Word Book*.

answer – and probably the origin of all philosophy – is to be found (as Jeeves used to remark) 'in the psychology of the individual.'

Three 'Radcliffe armchair lectures'[2]

There are times – the first working day after Christmas being one of them – when the academic life beckons most beguilingly. Its more elevated strata, at any rate. Being a Professor, say. Those long holidays so essential for restoring one's intellectual edge. The round of conferences pushing back the frontiers of knowledge with colleagues in the sunnier parts of the world. Leisurely strolls of an afternoon through the pastures of Journal-land, carving another notch on the walking stick for every mention of one's own name in a reference or footnote. After tea, (should the flow of publications bearing one's name have briefly wobbled), a spell of whip-cracking amongst the beavering ranks of one's Junior Lecturers known outside the Department as 'et al.'

Until now, these my petty jealousies have been no more than pipe dreams. Oxford may have its Regius Professor of Medicine, and 'Good luck, Reg,' say I. Margaret Thatcher may have her Personal Chair in Social Integration Studies at the University of Life, and I say, 'Well, if the seat fits …' But robes and deference are not my destiny. My lot has been to stand well back from the kerb as the academic juggernauts splash unheeding through the puddles of scholarship. Until now.

For the best part of a decade the proprietors of the Green Journal have allowed me the freedom of its columns to gesticulate from the sidewalk under a book-reviewer's flag of convenience. That period now over, and just as I was contemplating the long dark invisibility of my remaining career, imagine my delight when the Editorial Board graciously proposed me for a Radcliffe Personal Armchair in Clinical Philosophy.

There comes a moment in a man's life when he must set upon his principles a price far higher than the accoutrements of earthly vanity. But this was not that moment. 'You do me too much honour,' quoth I, and signed swiftly on the dotted line.

First among the official duties of a new Professor is to deliver The Inaugural Lecture. Traditionally this is an occasion for setting out one's stall, Sellotaping one's colours to the mast, and allowing a tantalising glimpse of work in progress which one has thoughtfully so far held back from publication. The professorial disquisition is sandwiched between two bits from the chairman, who is required to open proceedings with an affecting but unrecognisable eulogy, and to close them immediately the lecture ends by saying, 'Well if there are no questions …' and whisking one off for a sherry. Now, I can stand any amount of obsequious sycophancy as long as it's genuine, but as an Armchair Professor I eschew the formal platform in favour of the written discourse, being something I can do sitting down. But what I *would* have said would have taken up three lectures, and they would have gone something like this …

---

[2] Reprinted with modifications from *Education for General Practice* (1999), **10**, 203–6; **10**, 320–4; and **10**, 527–9.

Lecture 1 – On contemplative research

My Lord Publisher, ladies, gentlemen, fellow toilers in the vineyard:

It's astonishing how many advances in our understanding of the universe have occurred as the result of something dropping.

The celestial bodies, as un-shipshape a bunch as anything outside Government, soon got their orbits sorted out once the apple had dropped on to Isaac Newton's head. Einstein's special theory of relativity was conceived (according to some historians) when the impecunious young genius and his last ten Swiss centimes were set in relative motion as the coin, falling from his grasp while he descended an escalator at Zurich station, disappeared into the gap between the treads. And so many things were let slip in Sigmund Freud's consulting room in Vienna that it's a mercy his psychoanalytic theories are quite so back-of-an-envelope simple.

In my own case, at the age of 16 and in order to do biology in the sixth form, I dropped Greek. My command of the language at the time already enabled me nonchalantly to inform any passing Spartan that 'the-Themistocles is sitting-as-suppliant on the of-the-goddess altar'. Nevertheless, my determination to 'do medicine' had not faltered since the day I broke the milkman's leg in a collision with my tricycle, and I hardened my teenage heart even against the lure of the aorist subjunctive. The Greek master, never one to give up easily, tried to entice me back out of the bilge lab by asking, first, if I agreed that the function of an intelligent mind was to make new discoveries; and secondly, (granted that I might so agree), whether I realised that the goal thus envisioned was that of Hippocrates, no less. 'Coo,' I said. 'Well there we are then,' said he, and left me, rather abruptly I thought, to continue my dissection of the branchial arches of the dogfish.

Thus was laid the path which – I leave out the decades of intervening detail – has brought me to this comfortably upholstered Armchair of Clinical Philosophy.

'And what,' I hear you ask, 'is the defining contribution of so cushy-sounding a discipline to the relief of human suffering?'

And I reply, 'Contemplative research.'

People who wish to be thought wise – amongst whom we must include the editors of learned scientific journals, but not the company of saints, mystics or the more enduring novelists – tell us that truth is to be extracted from Nature by the application of certain forms of torture which we call research.

Conventional research comes in two kinds. Akin to the drip-drip of the Chinese water torture is *quantitative research*, much admired by sadists for the way it brings the cosmos to its knees by denying it sleep and thus sapping its will to remain secret. The other is *qualitative research*, a less sophisticated method resembling the rack, whereon Creation is stretched a little and threatened with more until it confesses to something the inquisitor knows already.

Enough of metaphor. There is at least one more way of interrogating the world, a gentler way, one that's not embarrassed sometimes to get things wrong, if that should be the price of sometimes getting things a different kind of right. That third way is *contemplative research*. We'll see how the three modalities interlock if we distinguish the separate questions each aspires to answer.

If I could have the first slide, please.

> ▨   Quantitative research asks, 'What is true?'

And the next.

> ▨   Qualitative research asks, 'What is interesting?'

And the next.

> ▨   Contemplative research asks, 'What matters?'

In other words, if you have ever thought that human values and priorities and assumptions should be – *are* – integral to deciding what we should enquire into, then you will incline towards contemplative research. If you've ever scanned the literature and found precious little you cared a toss about, no article you'd dream of reading if it was just you and the journal on a desert island, then you are a contemplative researcher at heart. If life would be all the sweeter if you never saw another correlation coefficient, Likert rating scale or semi-structured questionnaire, and yet you sincerely believed that nothing is more worthy of human endeavour than to see if things make sense, then your preferred research tool may yet be the armchair.

Think of it this way. Both qualitative and quantitative research deliver 'bottom-up' views of reality. They focus on small component parts and how they articu-late one with another, trusting that in time the big picture will become discernible. Contemplative research, by contrast, is 'top-down'. Contemplative researchers say to themselves, 'That would be a good thing to have a picture of; let's see what we'd need in order to create one. That's an important problem; let's see what might be getting in the way of understanding it. That's an interesting idea; but I wonder what evidence would look like.'

Is this all sounding a bit theoretical? Let's take a historical example of a first-class contemplative researcher in action – Charles Darwin. The American philosopher Daniel Dennett has called Darwin's 'natural selection' hypothesis 'the single best idea anyone has ever had … a universal acid, eating through every traditional concept, leaving a revolutionised world-view, transforming psychology, politics, ethics and religion'. The outline of Darwin's story will probably be familiar: the 22-year-old naturalist sailing for South America in 1831 aboard the *Beagle*; the qualitative studies of fossilised mammalian bones in Argentina; the quantita-tive observations of the differences between the finches and tortoises of the mainland and those on the Galapagos islands; the crystallising of insight on read-ing Malthus' essay on population growth; the further decade of pre-publication anxiety, fearing the scorn and ostracism which he thought his 'anti-religious' evolutionary notions would earn him.

In hindsight, which is most researchers' preferred way of writing up their work, the conclusions appear to arise logically and unambiguously from the data. The fossil record shows us *this*; observations of animal behaviour show us *that*; *ergo*, we infer a law that says the fittest survive. But the process of creative discovery wasn't like that. The evidence would have stood other interpretations, such as that God created a misleading fossil record in order coyly to cover His tracks. The unanswered questions clamour. Why was *this* the trip that Darwin chose to undertake? Why were *these* the fossils and *these* the species that took his attention? Why was it for Charles Darwin, of all people, that finding an explanation for life's diversity became a lifetime's quest, even at the risk of calumny and ridicule?

Darwin was a martyr to sea-sickness, and spent much of his time at sea whimpering in a hammock with his eyes closed. At such nauseous times one's past life lurches before one in bilious waves. He'd have remembered, pale-faced, dropping out of medical school in Edinburgh after two years, his father's ambition for him to become a doctor drowned out by the screaming of the surgical patients. Only individuals with a certain kind of fitness could have survived it. Three years of boredom at Cambridge before dropping his father's alternative career sugges-tion, divinity, would have confirmed that he was by nature ill-selected for such a course. Within reach would have been the copy of Lyell's *Principles of geology* – 'the face of the Earth has changed gradually over aeons through eruptions, earthquake and erosion' – dropped into his hand by his mentor John Henslow, as the *Beagle* weighed anchor, with the injunction, 'Read this, but don't believe it.'

You get the drift. If we want to understand what brought Darwin to the threshold of one of civilisation's greatest insights, the answer doesn't lie, even in principle, solely in qualitative or quantitative research. The third dimension, con-templative research, was necessary – private, eyes-closed-in-a-hammock research into how far a rebellious nature might go in questioning the assumptions of a 'father knows best' world-view, research that wondered what analogies and metaphors might productively be examined between the living and the non-living worlds, and dared to ask what idiocies might go unchallenged simply because they come with the Church's imprimatur.

Contemplative research takes as its starting point the gap between aspiration and attainment, the problems we long to solve and yet which stubbornly refuse to yield to the best analysis we have so far come up with. Contemplative research reveals that the gap often arises not from lack of facts but from inadequacies of mind-set.

There is, I shall be maintaining, an inner world of beliefs and values, habits and assumptions, myths and fallacies, ambitions and prejudices in which the fragile facts of scientific truth must struggle to secure a foothold of acceptance. This is indeed a Darwinian struggle. Whatever versions of 'truth' survive do so only insofar as they are harmoniously adapted to this inner world. We are to imagine qualitative and quantitative research as throwing up innumerable species of truth, with our own all-too-human foibles then tending to select out all but the most comfortable. But where truth is concerned, comfortable does not always mean best. We have the power, not least through philosophical conjecture, to change the intellectual environment that acts on our emerging ideas so as to favour such characteristics as balance, honesty, helpfulness, cooperation and common sense.

Contemplative research carries out its field work wherever people believe, with the greatest possible self-deluding sincerity, that they are engaged with the greatest possible wisdom and from the loftiest possible motives upon some-thing important. Contemplative research gathers its data, and studies how people behave, in committee rooms, or in the corridors of political power, or in seminar rooms and lecture theatres where the old-and-therefore-wise try to control the evolution of the young-and-therefore-ignorant.

You, a mainly medical audience, will quickly appreciate that contemplative research is a discipline where you will feel very much at home. I suspect many of you are already skilled in one of its core investigative procedures, retrospective icteroscopy – looking at things in hindsight through a jaundiced eye.

'Oh it's mere cynicism, is it?', I hear someone cry. Yet there is nothing 'mere' about cynicism in a clinical context. Naïveté is far more dangerous. Anyway, what else is a cynic, if not a passionate idealist who happens to be agonisingly shy?

In my second lecture I'll present some of contemplative research's early results in the form of axioms, aphorisms and laws, for you to test in the laboratory of your own inner sense. But to summarise:

> *What we know is governed by how we come to know it.*
>
> *What we can discover is limited by, and depends upon, the way we choose to look for it.*
>
> *The process of discovery is a reflection and projection of the inner mental processes of the researcher.*

See you next time.

Lecture 2 – Axioms, laws and the VIPERS engine

I met a real-life clinical philosopher once. Okay, so it *was* in Chicago and his name was Reisenschein or some such. But he was on the staff at one of the city's main hospitals, and he had a white coat and a space with his name on in the parking lot. I was there at a conference, strutting my stuff as the consultation know-all from the Old Country. In the bar after my session, we got talking about patient autonomy, which in the USA is synonymous with the ability to pay for treatment and in the UK with the right *not* to.

And then his bleep went off. He carried a bleep. Dr Reisenschein was the *on-call* clinical philosopher. Only in America.

It transpired there'd been a philosophical emergency in the Emergency Room. A drunken realtor from Winnetka had thrown up over a pregnant native American; her partner had clocked him one, and a dispute had arisen over who had the priority claim on the services of the on-call lawyer. Only in America, unfortunately. In Britain they'd have found a way to blame the GP. My new friend – and how proud Wittgenstein would have been of him – persuaded them to discard pre-conceived constructions that distinguish between consciousness and the external world, the utilitarian concept of *Zuhandsein* or 'being-at-hand' being epistemologically prior to the objectivised conception of *Vorhandsein* or 'being-on-hand'. She the puked-over was all for an inauthentic retreat into the communal anonymity of *Mitwelt*, which obviously would have reduced the self and others to on-hand existents. But the men thought a McDonalds was a better idea, so the whole thing ended happily.

It made me think. It concerned me that issues of right and wrong had become so far divorced from clinical practice, so marginalised from real doctoring, that they ended up being dumped on to some poor over-qualified bleep-slave who would otherwise have been emptying garbage bins. But at least they *had* one. Some hospital appointments board had deliberated, drawn up a job description, advertised, interviewed. And somewhere out in down-town Chicago at least one morally literate person had seen the ad, reckoned 'That's for me', and was now giving it his best shot. Us, we'd go all British at the very idea. Shame on us.

I don't know whether it's uplifting or just terrifying, but sometimes even the most random of experiences can slap you in the face with one of life's eternal verities. Watching amused as Dr Reisenschein scurried off on his errand of philosophical mercy, his on-call bag seemingly full of nothing but inanities, the goose-bumps on my neck nevertheless told me I was in the presence of a fundamental law of the Universe. In the sixth century BC the Taoist philosopher Lao Tsu put it this way:

> *See simplicity in the complicated.*
> *Achieve greatness in little things.*
> *In the universe the difficult things are done as if they are easy.*
> *In the universe great acts are made up of small deeds.*
> *Because the sage always confronts difficulties,*
> *He never experiences them.*

Or, as we might say nowadays, more succinctly, 'There's always *one.*'

And that one shouldn't just be Dr Reisenschein. It should be *us.*

Some wag – probably a Government Minister caught *in flagrante* – once remarked, 'Life is too big for the small questions.' I disagree. Life's usually too small for the big ones. Philosophy has ready answers for trifling little questions like, 'What's the purpose of existence?' But then, so does a child of six; the answer's easy-peasy – a Mars bar, or a game of Super-Cosmic Alien-Blasters. Naïve common sense will carry us thus far. No, it's the *big* questions we need philosophers for, questions such as, 'Why, two times out of five, does the last patient of the day get up my nose? But send me home rejoicing the other three times?'

Okay then, I hear you mutter. What *is* the purpose of existence? Is it deducible from first principles? What *are* 'first principles', the ones that have to be acknowledged as true *a priori*? Does contemplative research have its own axioms and laws and theorems, capable of reaching the parts that matter in professional life without our having to abandon the comfort of our own armchairs for the tiresomeness of actual experimentation?

And well, yes it does. Simple questions – sadly – tend to have complicated answers, and simple solutions – foolishly – tend to get applied to complicated problems. Complicated questions – luckily – often turn out to have been simple after all, but not before simple but wrong answers have been tried. It seems that, just as nature abhors a vacuum, human nature can only stand so much simplicity.

This in fact is a fundamental law discovered by contemplative research – the *Law of Constant Complexity*. First slide please.

> ▦ *Law of Constant Complexity*
>
> If one part of a closed complex system is made more simple, another part will become correspondingly more complicated.

We see this law at work in committees and task forces, when, typically, an apparent breakthrough or moment of clarity emanating from one member is immediately negated or obfuscated by someone else. Just when you think you've cracked a tricky problem, there's always someone who'll pipe up, 'That's all very well, but ...'

The Law of Constant Complexity has the following corollary, which I call *Resolution Paralysis*.

> ▦ *Resolution Paralysis*
>
> If a problem appears to be nearing solution, the number of points of view to consider will increase until insolubility is restored.

The principle underlying Constant Complexity and Resolution Paralysis is pure Darwinism. From the point of view of the *'species'* (committee, organisation, Department), making simple things complicated has survival value. The group task is never accomplished, therefore the group must continue indefinitely. At the level of the *individual* member of the group, this imperative translates into making things just sufficiently complicated that only oneself can understand them; thus one can never be dispensed with.

Anyway, let's apply a little contemplative research to the old 'meaning of life' conundrum. Next slide, please.

> ▦ *Axiom*
>
> The goal of all living systems is to prevail.

Obviously; if it wasn't, we'd all be dead. Or enlightened.

The phrase 'living systems' encompasses more than just biological organisms. You will probably accept, albeit secretly, that we humans are each ambitious on behalf not just of our genes but also of our reputation, our role, our self-image, our influence. We carry (in Robert Ardrey's phrase) our 'territorial imperative' into many arenas – family, committee room, polling booth, tutorial, surgery. And though we might shrink from dignifying them with the label 'instincts', we each experience territorial urges to compete, to dominate, to smother, to control, to recruit, to attack, to overwhelm, to besiege, to starve out, to see off. In a word, to win. I know, it makes us sound beastly, and of course we can offset the nastier side of our natures with lots of goodness and kindness and all the cuddlier ways of prevailing. But there we are. That's the biological part of our inheritance, and we're stuck with it.

Psychologists tell us that what we subjectively experience as motivation is actually a signal, alerting us to the presence of an unmet need. Low blood sugar? – you need more food, so eat! Low self-esteem? – you're under-achieving, so sign up for another course. Poor self-image? – find yourself a new role.

The fact is, we're always feeling motivated in one direction or another. While the world as a whole contains abundance of opportunity for all, no one person ever admits for long to having enough. To the individual's way of thinking, there always seems to be an excess of need over provision, an excess of entitlement over resources, of ambition over opportunity, of restraint over freedom, of unfairness over justice. We could even derive a general law, the *Law of Perpetual Shortfall.*

> ▩ *Law of Perpetual Shortfall*
>
> Individuals always perceive there to be a local shortage of resources.

This law creates an ever-available role, always there for the playing whenever things aren't ideal – the role of *Victim*. Wherever there's life, there's a Victim. Low blood sugar? – I'm the victim of hunger. Low self-esteem? – I'm a victim of Society. Low self-image? – I'm the victim of my upbringing.

By the same token, for things to get better, someone or something has to be got the better of. Not *us*, though. If someone's got to be the loser, we'd rather it was someone else. And so, if we're unlucky enough to find ourselves in a Victim role, we convince ourselves that it's because there is someone out there in the complementary role of *Persecutor*. If I scrape the car, it's because some idiot stuck a bollard in the way. If I fail an exam, it's because the examiners don't know quality when they see it. If I'm having a bad day at work, it's because the patients are unreasonable. Moreover, it's not always other people who are cast in the Persecutor role. It can be a thing, or an idea. Fate. Sod's law. The system. The regulations. The sexual revolution. The weather. The Lottery. The virus that's going about. At all events, wherever there's a Victim we'll find – or invent one if we have to – a Persecutor.

Is this all there is to life, existence only a two-state condition, the play on the world stage a budget two-hander featuring only Victim and Persecutor? Are we condemned to be either predator or prey, villain or patsy, forever toggling between the two, sometimes winning, other times losing, kicking or being kicked? No indeed. The repertoire of human interaction is more extensive. There is at least one more role available, that of *Rescuer*. This is a consequence of a universal fallacy which I call *The Egocentric Aberration*. Let me explain.

Einstein's theories of relativity include the apparently preposterous notion that 'Space is curved in the vicinity of mass'. What does that mean? Suppose you're a little ray of sunshine pootling through the universe the only way you know how, in a dead straight line. Suddenly someone sticks a dirty great lump of rock on your starboard beam, so close you could nearly touch it. What do you do? Well you swerve, don't you? You veer slightly towards the said lump of rock; you alter course a fraction and then continue on a heading just a bit to the right of previous. This of course is in flagrant breach of all accepted laws, which forbid little rays of sunshine to be diverted by anything at all. 'Not guilty,' you protest. 'It was the rock's fault. It curved my space like the camber on the A41 south of Aylesbury. I steered straight, but the road wobbled me.'

Well, mental life is a bit like that. Think of some of the laws we take for granted, and which you can see operating even-handedly and with 100% probability on everybody else. The law of averages. The laws of chance and diminishing returns. The laws of the jungle and of supply and demand. The Road Traffic Act and the Vocational Training Regulations 1997; Parkinson's law, and Murphy's; and that rather disagreeable one about all flesh being as grass. Somewhere in the small print of all of them, we are convinced, is an exclusion clause that says, 'But it doesn't apply to *me*.' The inevitabilities that apply to other people make a swerve around *me*. I'm an exception. In other words:

▦ *The Egocentric Aberration*

Probability is curved in the vicinity of oneself.

We try to reconcile (on the one hand) the laws of cause and effect as we see them applying to other people with (on the other) the psychological conviction that they shouldn't have to apply to *us*. And, primitive creatures that we are, the only way we can square the circle is by calling into being a *Rescuer* with the power to sort things out for us. Finding oneself in a Victim role prompts two reactions. The first is to nominate a Persecutor to lay the blame on; the second, to identify, in reality or in the imagination, a potential Rescuer. God used to have a monopoly on the Rescuer role, but it's been privatised. Nowadays the franchise is shared among doctors, politicians, lawyers, therapists. The pharmaceutical industry. Anybody, really. Social workers. In somebody's eyes, we can all be a hero, the Lone Ranger on the white horse. And it's rather fun. Playing the Rescuer sure beats being poor little Victim or villainous Persecutor.

Those of you who've read a bit of Transactional Analysis[3] will recognise in all this Karpman's 'Drama Triangle', in which the players of psychological games switch between the roles of Victim, Persecutor and Rescuer, scoring points off each other as they go. The analysis I've presented here acknowledges Karpman's description[4] and prepares the ground for applying it to wider contexts. The terms lend themselves to a nice little acronym – VIPERS, from VIctim, PErsecutor and ReScuer. As people endlessly circulate among these roles, they become the moving parts of the 'VIPERS engine', a three-stroke perpetual motion machine that imparts rotational energy to human affairs.

---

[3] Transactional Analysis: a school of analytic psychotherapy developed by Eric Berne. His fundamental model of the person is of having three 'ego states' – Parent, Adult and Child. Berne's best-known book is *Games people play* (1964) Grove Press, San Francisco.

[4] Karpman SB (1968) Fairy tales and script drama analysis. *Transactional Analysis Bulletin*, VII, **26**, 39–43.

In my next lecture I'll be examining some applications of the VIPERS engine, and taking another look at that unpleasantness involving St George and a dragon. In the meantime, I fancy I smell sherry beyond that green baize door. So, if there are no questions, I thank you for your attention, and look forward to seeing you again soon.

Lecture 3 – On dragons

Welcome back for the final 'armchair lecture' in this series.

Last time, I used the principles of contemplative research to derive a version of Karpman's Drama Triangle. Every player of life's great game, it transpires, can be cast in one of three roles – Victim, Persecutor or Rescuer. (From now on, let's indicate whichever role someone happens to be in at a given moment as VI, PE or RS.) 'As people endlessly circulate among these three', I said, 'they become the moving parts of the "VIPERS engine", a three-stroke perpetual motion machine that imparts rotational energy to human affairs.' So where do the dragons come in? Let me explain.

One warmish Spring Tuesday, in the year of our Lord two hundred and some-odd, young George of Cappadocia donned his shiniest armour and, sporting his favourite scarlet cross, mounted his trusty steed and went for a burn-up through the southern outskirts of the Libyan town of Sylene. As the *Sylene Messenger* subsequently reported, St George (for 'twould be he) chanced upon a horrendous scene.

There before his startled gaze, a horrid fiery dragon, all scales and bad breath, is about to blow-torch the milk-white skin off a chained damsel, with all the gusto of Gary Rhodes finishing off his *crèmes brûlées*. The *Messenger*'s chief reporter later penned an in-depth background piece. The dragon, it seems, was a distant cousin of Cetus the sea-monster, whom Perseus in days of yore had despatched for harbouring unchaste thoughts in respect of the fair princess Andromeda. The Sylene dragon, similarly disrespectful, had apparently issued an ultimatum to the effect that, unless pursuant to clauses etcetera etcetera a regular human sacrifice was provided on the terms set out in Appendix A, it would scorch the nuts off all townsfolk under the age of a hundred and twelve. Said sacrifice to be determined by ballot. List of candidates in said ballot to include the daughter of the king. Said princess now finds herself in bridal finery chained to the sacrificial rock, and said dragon, at the moment we pick up the story, finds itself squarely in the cross-wires of George's trusty lance. He charges; he engages; and a few pows, bams and splats later, the princess is free and our hero is leading the defeated dragon back to town on the end – and we won't enquire too closely – of the princess's girdle.

All perfectly straightforward in VIPERS terms, it would seem. The princess (VI) is rescued from the wicked dragon (PE) by the heroic knight (RS). Hoorah. End of story.

But. If Hollywood has taught us nothing else, we know that every story has its prequel and its sequel, its back-story and its next instalment, in which the unexpected happens and the roles are no longer what we assume them to be. In this case, for instance, our Sylene correspondent reports that George concluded his triumphal procession by announcing to the townsfolk that yes, certainly, he would kill the captured dragon for them – on condition that the entire population (some 15 000 souls) agreed to be converted to Christianity. Now I ask you; is *that* the action of a through-and-through hero? At a stroke the roles are recast. By imposing conditions, George, for all his noble intent, now becomes the Persecutor and the citizens (previously happy enough, for all we know, in their non-Christian state) are now the Victims of his blackmail. The poor old dragon must forfeit his life, not for any absolute good but in order that George may further his own personal agenda. Booo!

Note how the VIPERS engine has turned. The dragon has moved from Persecutor to a brief spell as Victim, and finally, in the sacrifice of death, to Rescuer; the Saint-to-be meanwhile has shifted from Rescuer to bullying Persecutor. The engine has exchanged its first Victim – the princess – for a fresh one, the community of reluctant converts. In the process, the destinies of all have been given a further spin and their careers a fresh momentum. And it doesn't end there.

George leaves town and rides off towards his eventual canonisation, his 'Rescuer' self-image intact unless at some future date he should find himself a potential Victim of either the dragon's big brother or a Sylenian priest of the old religion. The princess becomes a castrating old maid (PE), spurning all suitors (the next generation of Victims) because they aren't a patch on the heroic George. Around the grave of the newly-martyred dragon a reactionary anti-Christian cult of dragon-worship springs up, its subversive adherents pledging themselves Rescuers of the Old Way. And it doesn't end there ...

... nor, indeed, did the story begin where we joined it. All the characters have their back-stories. Maybe the dragon wasn't really a Persecutor. Maybe it had an unhappy childhood, its mother dead, its father a former Cabinet minister, its nanny a slipper-wielding transvestite. It just couldn't help itself (VI). Or perhaps (RS) it was a secret agent of the king all the time, the self-sacrificing instrument of a cunning royal plan to elevate the ugly unmarriageable princess to celebrity status in the hope of attracting the affections of knightly suitors.

And maybe the princess wasn't quite the luckless innocent she's made out to be. I suspect that, bored silly by her chaste and obedient life up at the palace, she'd secretly done a course on veterinary psychopathology and been to a workshop on counselling, and saw in the fortuitous arrival of the dragon a chance to act out some childhood domination fantasies under the guise of doing therapy on the unsuspecting beast. 'Doing therapy', as we all know, is an acceptable banner under which all manner of would-be Rescuers can march. It can also, as Ivan Illich, Thomas Szasz and R D Laing have pointed out, be a cover story for a particularly insidious form of psychological oppression. So the situation upon which George happened to chance was not the B-movie 'endangered moll' scenario, but rather the set-up for an elaborate emotional game between two consenting, though not fully informed, adults. Far from requiring the intervention of this unexpected and pushy knight, all the princess had to do (as we say nowadays) to 'achieve closure' was to take the dragon's £5 or pass him the Kleenex. In this version it's George who, by spoiling the princess's sport, unwittingly becomes her Persecutor.

Let's now contemplate all this research evidence in the laboratory of our armchair and see what conclusions it leads to, what hypotheses it suggests, and what on earth practical use it might be to anybody.

Most importantly, let's ask ourselves, 'Does it ring true?' Is this George/dragon/princess story so accurate an analogy, so universal a metaphor for some aspect of the human condition that we should afford it the dignity of an archetype?

I reckon so. But don't take my word for it: check it out in the familiar professional setting of the consulting room.

As a static description, the 'dragon' story fits the traditional medical model just fine. The patient (princess, Victim) is afflicted by a disease (dragon, Persecutor), and the doctor (George, Rescuer) cures it. The analogy holds even if we pursue it to the second stage of the mythical version: the heroic doctor, restoring the patient to her loved ones, basks in popular adulation, which he turns to his own and his profession's advantage by demanding substantial money and esteem as the price for continuing the noble work.

A key feature of the 'dragon' model, however, is the notion that, while a given story-line contains all three VIPERS roles, the roles are not fixed, neither are they always what they seem. Dragons don't always breathe fire, and the man on the white charger isn't always the hero. Each character, moreover, can play any of the three roles; every actor brings to *one* role a history of rehearsal in both the others, and may 'flip' during the course of the performance. Victims can turn into Persecutors, and Rescuers can find themselves recast as Victims. In the consulting room, the patient can turn into a heart-sink Persecutor, so that the doctor feels like the Victim. The disease, as ticket of admission or safety-valve for relieving stress, was the patient's real Rescuer all the time; and, if that particular Rescuer is removed, a new one must be found, possibly in the form of an out-patient referral or a Balint group.

A strong sense of perpetual motion emerges from this model, of individuals endlessly revolving around the three roles and, through their engagements with other people in other contexts, transmitting rotational energy one to another like a train of gears. If there are universal engines that drive human affairs, maybe this is one of them. It would be nice to think the VIPERS engine was the power source for some of our proudest achievements – the abolition of slavery, say, or the setting up of the NHS. I suspect, however, that most of what it causes is trouble – anxiety, bickering, frustration, buck-passing, grid-locked committees, dragged-out decision-making, planning blight, the Irish question.

If it really is role rotation that drives all these 'here we go again' scenarios, it would be nice to know either how to make the VIPERS engine run smoother, or else sometimes how to put so much grit in its bearings that it grinds to a halt. What sets the wheels in motion in the first place? Where's the brake? Have we any control over who takes what role? Is there a red button we can press if we get accidentally trapped in the moving machinery? My Department of Contemplative Research is actively working on these questions, and I hope to share some of our provisional findings with you in due course.

Unless, of course, some dragon gets me first.

On the tango[5]

As a limpet on a camel, so are you likely to find me on the dance floor. It's the body-work I can't get the hang of; it just seems so much algebra for the limbs. When the music starts I immediately make an inhibition of myself, developing a paralysis so complete that bystanders look around to see who fired the curare dart.

---

[5] *Behind the lines*, Back Pages, *Brit. J. Gen. Pract.*, June 2003.

I suppose I could always learn. Trouble is, my learning style's against me. By nature, I'm one of those cerebral types who like to grasp the concepts and master the theory before attempting a new skill. It's pathetic: my shelf of golf instruction manuals is as long as my handicap. But you'll perhaps understand why it was with mixed curiosity and trepidation that I opened a recent *BMJ*[6] and found it was a special themed edition devoted to − dancing.

Of course, being the *BMJ*, they dressed things up a bit. Not for them the diagrammed sequences of black and white footprints, or coy references to 'the lady and the gentleman'. Here, the dancing partners were designated 'doctors' and 'managers', and the key teaching point was this − it takes two to tango. But why a special edition? Well apparently, whereas doctors and managers as individuals and in the separate privacies of their own professional worlds can be lovely little movers, they've recently started going out together, and things aren't looking good in the dancing department. Initial sorties by the doctor-manager combo on to the sprung floor of the Healthcare Delivery Ballroom have been characterised by unseemly fumbling, clumsy footwork and some very bruised toes.

The problem, it seems, is that doctors think managers all have two left feet, and managers think doctors all have two right ones. Or, as the *BMJ* puts it, there is 'mutual distrust, personal abuse and blame', the protagonists having 'differing world views, steeped in historical rivalries that resurface at each encounter'. This should surprise nobody; managers cannot afford to become preoccupied with the needs of an individual patient irrespective of the consequences for others, while doctors can't put pre-ordained policy above the interests of the patient in front of them. We are all familiar with the attrition in the stand-off between medical and management value systems − the silly targets, the runaway drug budgets, the phoney waiting list statistics, the Newspeak redefinitions of things like quality, effectiveness, choice and care.

The solution, eloquently elaborated by the *BMJ*'s team of dance tutors, is also familiar. Doctors and managers need to quit behaving like prima ballerinas and start hoofing it as a proper twosome. It would be easy to cringe at the clichéd banalities in which this injunction is couched − 'constructive dialogue', 'inter-disciplinary education', 'working towards the alignment of mission and strategy'. Easy, but wrong; for (we are told) 'only a well functioning relationship can deliver real service improvements'.

Uh-oh. Did you clock the 'only'? An 'only' like that usually means someone is trying to slip a fallacy past you disguised as a truism. But surely no one could quibble with a call for doctors and managers to stop playing games and start relating like adults? Yet a fallacy there is.

Playing games? Relating like adults? Where have you heard this before? Of course − Eric (*Games people play*) Berne's Transactional Analysis, with its devastatingly insightful depiction of the human psyche as a Parent-Adult-Child triad. In a refinement of Berne's model, Stephen Karpman described a 'drama triangle'[7], where the players of psychological games rotate around the roles of Victim, Persecutor and Rescuer, scoring points off each other as they go. (Doctors and managers will smile a guilty smile of recognition.) A corollary of Karpman's

---

[6] *BMJ*, vol. 326, 22 March 2003. Subsequent quotations are from editorials and articles in this issue.
[7] Karpman SB (1968) Fairy tales and script drama analysis. *Transactional Analysis Bulletin*, VII, **26**, 39−43.

analysis is that when two parties are in unstable role equilibrium, *cherchez la troisième*. And who is the unseen third dancer, neither the deliverer of health care nor its organiser? Why, the policy maker! The politician. Add 'politician' to the dyad of doctor and manager, and (although there may be squabbling over who plays which of the three roles) Karpman's triangle takes on a terrifyingly accurate verisimilitude.

And where are the politicians, the draughtsmen of the big picture, in the *BMJ* analysis? Nowhere; not a single mention; air-brushed out. They are the Teflon tribe, to whom no responsibility may be seen to stick. They have control without involvement, power without experience. Their accountability to the electorate is, compared with doctors' vulnerability to complaint and that of managers to performance review, occasional and perfunctory.

So let us call for our politicians too to stop playing games with the NHS and get involved like responsible adults, on an equal footing with the other two parties. Come and join the dance. It would be an unfamiliar sight doctors, managers and politicians, arms linked and high-kicking. But this much I know about dancing: it takes three to tango.

On parsnips and quantum mechanics[8]

As I write, it's early Tuesday afternoon and I'm worried. I've just got back from lunch in the departmental canteen where I found (and the hairs on the back of my neck stand up again even as I recall it) that the boiled parsnips had butter on them. Canteen parsnips are usually presented to a hungry world garnished with a greyish dusting of fine volcanic ash, or just occasionally smeared with margarine. Once, after a recent visit from the Health and Safety people, they came drizzled with Benecol. But today they were (and there's only one word for it) swimming in (and there's only one word for it) – butter.

This can only spell trouble. It means that Carmen, our formidable maîtresse d', is Seriously Peeved. In the Department of Clinical Philosophy's staff canteen, buttered parsnips are like a coded message from the IRA, a warning that someone has been out-verballed and doesn't intend to take it lying down. And it can only be a response to yesterday's little unpleasantness.

Yesterday lunchtime, as I joined the slow lane snaking its way towards the non-stew option, I noticed Greg my Junior Lecturer enter the canteen in earnest conversation with Tamsin from Finance and Applied Uncertainty. Peeping out from above the zip of his anorak was the black and white face of a kitten, mewing with a piteousness usually associated with babies in the immunisation clinic, or their parents. 'Oh sweetums, what's its name?' Tamsin was asking, and Greg said, 'Schrödinger.' Tamsin said, 'As in ...' and Greg said, 'Exactly', and, laughing, they wagged fingers at each other in a get-the-in-joke kind of way.

Lost in their private world, Greg and Tamsin so far forgot their Britishness as to barge straight to the front of the queue, causing several colleagues who had been pressing forward with the intoxicating scent of macaroni cheese in their nostrils to fall backwards like a row of dominoes. One or two of them pursed their lips, and I heard someone mutter 'Really!' But Carmen – . I can hardly credit her recklessness;

---

[8] Reprinted from *Education for General Practice* (2001), **12**, 228–32.

I mean, you'd have thought that even an intelligence as unique as hers would have known that there's one thing you should never, ever say to a junior philosopher if he is the only thing standing between twenty-five other hungry philosophers and the dish of the day. But Carmen, with ladles akimbo, looked Greg in the eye, sniffed just once, and said it.

'Oi,' she said, 'what's the big idea?'

This produced an effect on Greg similar to that seen in about AD 30 when on a mount near Galilee someone asked our Lord whether by any chance he happened to have such a thing as a packed lunch for 5000 anywhere about him.

'The Big Idea,' echoed Greg, the light of Messianic fervour shining in his countenance. 'Thank you so much for asking. I will share with you the Big Idea, share it with *all* of you, share it now. Gather round.' And, with the exception of a few brave souls who saw which way the cookie was crumbling and sneaked off for a tuna bap at Lunchy-Munchies, gather round we did.

I'll say this for Greg — in many respects he's got the makings of a great teacher. The content is all there, as is enthusiasm, recognising the student's educational needs, plus spotting a chance for opportunistic learning and grabbing it by the throat. All he really lacks is a sense of the time and the place.

What follows is no more than a précis of the extempore tutorial that Greg then gave, the fallout from which I fear we are not done with yet.

'The Big Idea, Carmen,' he began, 'is quantum mechanics, and in particular quantum mechanics as applied to general practice. The big idea is to discover how the strange, irrational and counter-intuitive world of the infinitesimally small correlates with the strange, irrational and counter-intuitive ways patients behave at the doctor's.'

'Me, I've had this 'flu that's been going around,' Carmen volunteered, blowing her nose on a tea-towel and dropping it absent-mindedly into the custard.

'Then you will understand at once the application of de Broglie's idea of wave/particle duality,' said Greg with evident glee. Carmen, not sure whether the mickey was being taken, pawed the ground like a bull sizing up a matador.

'In experiments, let me remind you, light sometimes behaves as if it is a wave phenomenon, and at others as if it is a stream of particles, or photons,' Greg continued. Quailing momentarily before Carmen's baleful glare, he turned round to the rest of us, who were trying surreptitiously to liberate a few cooling sausages from their tray on the serving counter. 'It's simply a special case of Niels Bohr's principle of complementarity.' 'Oh absolutely,' we muttered shiftily.

Greg was getting into his stride. Although 'wave behaviour' and 'particle behaviour' would appear in theory to be mutually exclusive, he explained, in fact both are necessary for full understanding. Whether or not something behaves as a particle or a wave depends on one's choice of apparatus for looking at it. 'This principle of complementarity applies to light, or electrons, or,' he went on, turning back to Carmen, 'to 'flu.' 'What?' she snarled.

''Flu is a viral illness, right?' Greg asked. 'Right,' said nearly half his audience. 'Wrong,' said Greg. ''Flu is an expression of somatic anxiety and an unconscious wish to return to a state of infantile dependency?' 'Right,' said nearly the other half. 'Wrong: 'flu is an imbalance of chi resulting from a blockage to the free flow of kidney energy through the chakras,' said Tamsin brightly.

'The point,' Greg continued hastily, 'is that 'flu is neither just a virus nor just a state of mind, nor, Tamsin, just an energy problem. It's all of them, all at the same time. Which you decide is the 'true' explanation depends on what assumptions you make about the nature of reality, on what you are prepared to accept as evidence, on the language you adopt to express your explanatory framework and on what questions you choose to ask the patient.'

At this point the kitten Schrödinger resumed his mewing and, with a wriggle, leapt from the confines of Greg's anorak into a dish of fillet of cod Duglère where, as if by reflex, Carmen ladled gravy over him. The outraged moggie, looking as much dead as alive, shot off and took refuge on top of a pallet of tinned peaches, washing himself with an expression of long-suffering disdain. 'Schrödinger, here kitty kitty,' Greg called, to no avail.

'Why do you call him Schrödinger?' Tamsin enquired. (There's always someone, isn't there, who can be relied upon to toss up the easy lob for the champ to smash out of the stadium.)

'After Erwin Schrödinger of Zurich, the famous physicist and philanderer,' Greg replied. And he continued his public seminar.

'Schrödinger in 1935, you will recall,' (and we of the chorus nodded sagely) 'was pretty unhappy at what was becoming the standard quantum theory explanation for seemingly random events, the so-called Copenhagen Interpretation.' We listened with grudging admiration as Greg elaborated. The Copenhagen Interpretation, it transpired, asserted that the state of a system at the atomic level could not be completely defined. The most that could be said was that it possessed only the potentiality to have certain values with certain probabilities – until, that is, someone makes a measurement, at which point potentiality vanishes and only one form of certainty carries on existing. Until the defining act of measurement, *all* possible alternatives states – yes, each and every one – are simultaneously present, or as the quantum theorists like to put it, 'the act of observation collapses the superposition of multiple wave functions into a single one.'

Erwin Schrödinger, apparently, for all that he was a cutting edge physicist, couldn't square this with common sense, and devised his famous thought experiment. In it, he imagined a live cat placed into a sealed box containing a radioactive source, a Geiger counter, a hammer and a glass bottle of cyanide. Things are so arranged that the Geiger counter is switched on for just long enough for there to be a fifty–fifty chance that an atom of radioactive material will decay, be detected, and trigger the hammer to smash the glass bottle and thus gas the cat. As long as the box is sealed, we have no way of telling whether the cat is alive or dead. Moreover, until we look inside, the whole experiment is governed by the Copenhagen rule that all possibilities are real as long as they remain unexamined. The cat is neither alive nor dead; it is both alive *and* dead simultaneously in some hybrid state of suspended animation. Only at the instant of opening the box do the superimposed wave functions representing live-ness and dead-ness collapse into one of the two alternative states, and reveal on which side of the grave the cat is to be found.

Schrödinger, bless his naïve cotton socks, thought this proof that life and death could co-exist was self-evidently nonsense, and hoped his thought experiment would put an end to the increasingly wild speculations of the quantum fraternity. 'Nonsense at the cat level proves nonsense at the quantum level' was roughly his argument. But not a bit of it: the idea of mutually exclusive alternatives occupying the same neck of the experiential woods rather took off. Even Einstein's famous rhetorical question, 'Does God play dice with the universe?', gets the perfectly serious answer, 'Don't know: let's toss a coin – heads He does, tails He doesn't.' All possibilities exist simultaneously until the action of a human experimenter rules out all but one, the one surviving option which we, the conscious observer, have through our own intervention brought into existence.

Carmen sneezed. 'What's this got to do with my 'flu?' she asked, ever the pragmatist.

Greg rubbed his hands like a man limbering up for the big finale.

'Getting 'flu sets you up to be the subject of an experiment, much as Schrödinger's unfortunate cat was,' he said. 'Once in the box, the cat is just as much alive as dead, until somebody opens the box to look.'

A careful listener might have discerned a low rumbling sound in the canteen, as of two dozen of the world's unlunched starting to make 'get on with it' noises.

Greg ploughed resolutely ahead. 'The parallel case is this,' he said. 'The subjective experiences of illness and health are often found in a superimposed condition. It's possible to feel "ill" while organically in perfect health, and to feel "well" while suffering from definite physical disease. When the virus strikes, you have the potential to say to yourself *either* "I'm a generally well person who happens to get the occasional illness, this being one of them," *or* "I'm a generally ill person who happens to get the occasional spell of health, this *not* being one of them." The doctor who interrogates you to determine the nature of your disease becomes the observer who, by the act of framing his enquiry, causes one possibility to vanish and the other to remain. In general terms, illness and health are latent and superimposed until, in a particular case, one or other is brought into existence by the act of an outsider – the doctor – assessing it.'

'There,' he ended with a flourish, 'that was worth missing lunch for, wasn't it?', and pandemonium broke out. My last recollection is of Carmen standing on a table, the kitten Schrödinger clutched to her bust like Cleopatra's asp, yelling, 'Fine words – but they butter no parsnips!' Hence today's culinary anomaly; the parsnips *grand luxe* are, I presume, what to Carmen's way of thinking passes for irony.

* * *

I fled to my professorial armchair and, closing my eyelids, entered the sanctuary of that philosophical laboratory which sceptics call a light doze. Not for the first time, I reflected that metaphor is a marvellous tool for helping us feel at home in unfamiliar, though not completely alien, realms. It has a terrible power simultaneously to illuminate, unsettle and provoke. Not that Greg's tutorial on 'the doctor as defining observer' was anything other than sound. And not for the first time, too, it occurred to me that virtually everything in life can be fashioned into a useful metaphor for the practice of medicine. Unfortunately, the converse seems equally true, namely, that virtually everything in the practice of medicine can be fashioned into a useful metaphor for life. Life and medicine seem destined to exist in a perpetual state of 'mutual metaphor', each an allegory for the other in equal measure. And in which case, isn't metaphor as a currency in serious danger of being devalued?

Thus I mused, and some inkling of a resolution dawned. Such understanding of the world as we humans are capable of is constrained by the functioning of the human mind in all its conditions and configurations. If it seems inconceivable that an electron should be in two places at once; if an unseen cat cannot possibly be alive and dead at the same time; if we can know only one thing about a subatomic particle, its position or its momentum but not both – perhaps these paradoxes are no more than glimpses over the perimeter fence that marks the limit of the territory within which our minds have over the aeons evolved to function. If rational thought sets foot outside the conceptual backyard to which evolution has adapted it, it runs every explorer's risk of vanishing without trace. Some questions, such as 'Does the Higgs boson exist?' or 'Why does the last patient of evening surgery when you're going to the theatre always burst into tears?', are beyond the range of rational analysis, and as sterile from the outset as an argument about the grammar of Esperanto. As Anton Zeilinger of Vienna University has recently proposed, since the fundamental quantum of information is the 'yes/no bit' – the 'either/or beyond which no detail may be discerned' – the human mind can resolve no question more subtle than can be answered with a single bit. The 'grain' of the human image of the universe is thus defined as no smaller than one bit; any phenomenon more subtle than this is inevitably distorted in the attempt to represent it.

If we try to take something from yesterday's fiasco which has left Greg, bless him, *persona non grata* in the catering division, it could be this. To preserve the maximum range of human potential, the defining observation which eliminates every alternative except one should be delayed as long as possible. The only good options are open ones. To be specific, medicine is best served by doctors whose instinct is to prefer delayed understanding rather than an early rush to scientific closure. We need doctors who are at least as comfortable with the metaphorical kind of truth as with the rational.

From here it is but a short step to some radical proposals for the medical curriculum. No one should be admitted to medical school, for instance, unless they have an arts or humanities subject at A-level. Medical students scoring in the top 10% of science-based exams should have to repeat the course until they do worse. All medical records should be written in verse. The number of diagnoses or decisions a doctor may make in a single day should be capped.

But I daydream: in the meantime there are the small matters of persuading Carmen to restore her parsnips to their pre-ironic state and of reminding Greg that Schrödinger is a cat, not a visual aid. Sometimes I wonder whether clinical philosophy is worth the effort. Brain surgery might be easier.

5

The case of the
blue-bottomed sheep

It started with an innocent little piece in the *Back Pages* in February 2002. I had spent Christmas with friends in Langholm, Dumfriesshire. The previous year had seen the British farming industry and countryside scourged by foot and mouth disease, so the appearance once more of sheep on the Scottish hills was cause for rejoicing. At the same time, Dr Andrew Wakefield's controversial suggestion of a link between MMR vaccine and childhood autism had blown immunisation targets out of the water, and everyone wanted to know whether little Leo Blair, the Prime Minister's youngest child and aged 19 months at the time, had had his MMR[1]. The connection seemed, if not obvious, at least worth exploring.

After the piece appeared, Alec Logan, the *Back Pages* editor, e-mailed me to dispute my use of the word 'tup' to mean a ram, and also what a ram loves doing. Confronted with dictionary evidence that I was right, Alec withdrew, but bet me a bottle of champagne that I couldn't weave a specified bunch of other meanings and spellings of the word into my next column. So naturally I accepted the challenge. The following month's piece, *On hypocrisy*, had them all in, and a few more besides. A magnum of non-vintage Veuve Clicquot Ponsardin Brut was my reward.

Then in January 2003 Alec e-mailed again. He had been given the *Cassell Dictionary of Slang* for Christmas, and had rushed to look up 'tup'. Four meanings were documented – 'a cuckold' (16th century); 'a very small amount' (mid-19th century); 'to arrest' (late-19th century); and 'to have sexual intercourse' (late-16th century). 'My challenge to you,' he wrote, sad man that he is, 'is to use 'tup' in all four senses of the word in the same column before June, and without seeming contrived or self-indulgent.'

Contrived or self-indulgent, *moi*? Naturally, sad man that I am, I accepted the challenge. The piece *On words* won me this time a bottle of vintage Krug, which Alec, I and James Willis (another frequent contributor to the *Back Pages*) consumed after the Annual General Meeting of the RCGP in November 2003 at which I was installed as President.

Doesn't it reassure you that the affairs of the Royal College and its prestigious Journal are in the hands of such gentlemen? No prizes for an answer.

---

[1] It was later alleged (*Sunday Times*, 29th February 2004) that Leo did indeed receive MMR vaccine – but not until he was more than 18 months old, three to six months later than the Department of Health recommends.

On sheep[2]

Christmas in the Scottish Borders. The clouds have broken their promise of snow and let down only a Presbyterian drizzle. In Dumfries and Galloway, finally free of foot and mouth disease, sheep are once more in evidence. The grass is lusher than usual, last season's growth left only half-nibbled by their slaughtered predecessors, with the stench of whose burning carcasses the air no longer reeks.

On the hillside above Langholm a small flock is grazing. And they have blue bottoms. The sheep's bottoms are – well, there's only one word for it – blue. Bright blue. My hostess is a former sex therapist with Relate and therefore qualified to advise on such intimate mysteries. It's only the ewes who have blue bottoms, she points out. The tups have had their tummies painted blue. She taps her nose knowingly, and the penny drops. During this the rutting season, the farmer has devised a contact-tracing strategy at whose effective simplicity the staff of every GUM clinic can only gasp in admiration. A blue bottom means 'recently serviced'.

On closer inspection, not all the ewes are equally committed to the cause of cerulean fundamentalism. A few appear to have signed a pledge of purity and still have their nethers undyed. These are the sheepish virgins, the Ann Widdecombes of the ovine world. On others, by contrast, the blue badge of congress is so vivid as to mark them out as ewes of easy virtue or *Playram* centrefolds. So far no tup looks to be sullied *a posteriori* with the tell-tale stain, but these are liberal times ...

Outraged, I feel an ethical protest is called for. To have one's sexual status colour-coded and flaunted for all to titter at makes a mockery of every principle of confidentiality. It's a disgraceful breach of the shepherd-sheep relationship, beside which all the recent hoo-hah about the public's right to know if the Prime Minister's youngest has had his MMR vaccine seems small beer.

Whether Leo Blair is jabbed or unjabbed matters less than his father's frantic attempts to avoid telling us which. The 'whether to immunise' decision is a private matter between Leo's parents and doctor, doubtless made after the fullest consideration of the facts and circumstances. But the 'whether to disclose' decision is another matter entirely, with genuine public repercussions. A College spokesman was quick off the blocks, harrumphing predictably about threats to the doctor-patient relationship, but addressing the wrong question. Whatever may have been threatened on this occasion – mainly a politician's inalienable right to conceal hypocrisy – it certainly wasn't the sanctity of the consulting room. As I recall, indeed, no member of the press had even considered the Blairs' GP as a potential mole or whistle-blower.

Mind you, I can't for the life of me think why not, given the ease with which some supposedly impregnable bastions of our ethical creed have crumpled in the face of the Government's secret weapon – cash.

I suspect someone in Whitehall is employed to maintain a current price list for the medical profession's principles. Do you doubt it? Then think of Ernest Bevan stopping the consultants' mouths with gold; remember Ken Clarke observing how GPs feel nervously for their wallets at the mention of reform. Recall how, more recently and more insidiously, we GPs have been systematically bribed into becoming enforcers of central policy. Fund-holding, PMS, prescribing incentive

---

[2] *Behind the lines*, Back Pages, Brit. J. Gen. Pract., February 2002.

schemes, new patient checks, smear and immunisation targets – what are these if not backhanders to encourage us, when push comes to shove, to overrule patient autonomy and renege on our advocacy of individual patients in favour of politically-imposed priorities? Oh sure, Government usually offers us a get-out clause, one of its range of Newspeak slogans, so that we can betray loyalties without too great a sense of guilt. We're not selling out to the Department of Health, we're 'adding a dimension of outcome-related incentivisation in social accountability'. Or something.

Bullshit. An increasing proportion of our income is tainted money, and it shouldn't be. But fear not: I have (like Jonathan Swift of old) a 'modest proposal' to restore moral consistency to our profession.

Patients who are up-to-date with their immunisations and smears, who maintain a cholesterol of less than five on diet alone, who promise not to join any waiting list longer than three months, and who keep the cost of their prescribed medication in the bottom quartile for their age will be designated 'beacon patients'. GPs who release the names of their beacon patients to the press, where they will be held up for public acclaim as an encouragement to others, will be paid £500 per patient.

Paid £500, and have their bottoms painted blue.

On hypocrisy[3]

In last month's *Back Pages*, I denounced as a breach of confidentiality the use by Scottish shepherds of blue paint to track the copulatory contacts between male sheep, or tups, and their lady flock-mates. The column prompted the following letter from a retired farmer in the Brecon Beacons.

'Sir,' he wrote, 'I beg to inform you that I found your article about tups to be Not At All Funny, and was the cause of words between myself and my lady wife, née Tupp. It has been my pleasure these many years to refer by jocularity to her brother the Reverend Gareth as "the tup-hog" and to Evan his first-born, our nephew, as "the tup-lamb". Even (may God forgive me due to stress) that barren ewe who is the wife's mother I call her "the tup-yeld". Your tip about the blue paint put me in mind of some malarkey to enliven the Tupperware parties to which my lady wife is much given, and am pending litigation ...'

No, I have to come clean. I had no such letter. It was make-believe – but invented for a reason I wish, gentle Reader, to confess to you.

On receiving my manuscript for the 'blue-bottomed sheep' piece, Alec the Editor had, (rather unfairly, I thought, he being a native Scot) queried my use of the word 'tup' on physiological grounds. He claimed that a toop, tuip or teep (as he variously spelt it, Scots being a no-go zone for the spell-check facility) had been castrated, and was therefore unable to rise to the occasion in the manner described. *The Concise Scots Dictionary* (Aberdeen University Press, p. 740) put him right, however; and Alec, gentleman that he is, pledged me a bottle of champagne if I incorporated into this column a specified selection of shepherding *patois* such as 'toop', 'tup-yeld' – I leave you to spot the others.

---

[3] *Behind the lines*, Back Pages, *Brit. J. Gen. Pract.*, March 2002.

Well they're all there, Alec. Put that in your tup-horn and blow it; I and my empty glass await our reward.

Nevertheless the exercise has confronted me with the price of my own honour. If it comes to a choice between prostituting my art as a columnist and a bottle of Krug '45, then it seems I'm for prostitution. It's worse than that: in last month's piece I was chastising our profession for its willingness to play Government's silly games for money, and now here am I . . .

So what sort of a hypocrite does this make me? Just the common or garden sort, I dare say.

It's part of being human sometimes to do good things, and sometimes bad; and to do them sometimes for good reasons, and sometimes for bad. To do good things for good reasons is the act of a saint or a lover, and relatively rare. To do bad things for bad reasons is also rare, rarer than the sanctimonious would have us believe. But most people lead their moral lives sloshing around in the middle, doing good things for bad reasons and bad things for good ones. We can – if we call it anything at all other than normal – call this paradox 'the human condition' to make ourselves feel better, but it's a passing fair definition of hypocrisy nonetheless.

One function of civilisation, it seems to me, is to contain our hypocrisies within an acceptable frame. The great professions exist to champion our greatest visions of what is good – health, wealth, justice, knowledge, security – while at the same time keeping our bad reasons for pursuing them – exploitation, greed, self-aggrandisement – within bounds.

That's a heavy responsibility, I reckon, to lay on the shoulders of any profession comprised of mortals, even, as in our own case, of medically qualified mortals. I suspect the only way individual professionals like you and me can cope with it is by allowing the big paradox, the big hypocrisy, the big inconsistencies to trickle down until, acceptably diluted, they seep all but imperceptibly into the fibre and fabric of our everyday practice. Hypocrisy on the small scale is our stock in trade. We believe in continuity of care until the phone rings at 3 am, and in personal doctoring until we go on a mid-week conference. Prescribing an antibiotic for a URTI doesn't seem as bad in a five-minute appointment as in a ten. Even our much-vaunted 'patient-centred consulting' can swiftly degenerate into simulation, a mere going through the motions of a *caritas* we often do not feel, yet dare not deny.

As grease in the professional workings, maybe a bit of judicious hypocrisy is no bad thing. If there was a vaccine against double standards, I doubt many doctors would have it.

So what sort of hypocrite has Alec's champagne trick shown me to be? A dyed-in-the-wool one, I guess. Am I alone?

On words[4]

'What's in a name?' asked the Bard of Avon (whose own name, you'll recall, was Shake-speare, not Wobble-spike, or even Wag-staff). 'That which we call a rose,' he asserted, 'by any other name would smell as sweet.'

---

[4] *Behind the lines*, Back Pages, *Brit. J. Gen. Pract.*, May 2003.

Possibly, and possibly not. Some early botanist, coming at it cold, might have chanced upon a previously unknown and unnamed species, breathed its dreamy fragrance, and exclaimed, 'Ah sweet flower, I shall call thee — zose.' And since the word 'zose' stood for nothing pre-existing, he might have got away with it. If my flower-beds were full of zoses, not roses, I'd be with Shakespeare and not give a fig for what particular syllables we used to refer to them. But had that long-dead bestower of names lit instead upon the word 'sprout', or 'belch' — you get my drift. The scent molecules hitting my olfactory epithelium might be the same, but tell me what I'm smelling is a sprout and I suspect the edge will be taken off my enchantment. What P G Wodehouse called 'the psychology of the individual' is at work. It doesn't matter what you call something, as long as what you call it doesn't have conflicting associations. But if it does, the name alters the experience.

Take another case in point: the word 'tup', another of Shakespeare's favourites. You might recall a while back (on page 46) I told you of the blue-bottomed sheep of Dumfries, whose newly-serviced sisters bore the tell-tale badge of deflowerment transferred from the blue-painted bellies of the rams (or 'tups') who had obliged ('tupped') them under cover of darkness. Now, veterinary sources confirm that tupping occupies less than 1% of a ram's working day, the rest being equally divided between eating grass and devising a proof of Fermat's Last Theorem. But note the usage; when 'tup' makes the transition from noun to verb, only one small part of the animal's skills repertoire is emphasised, and that salaciously. And so when, in *Othello*, Iago tells Desdemona's father that 'an old Blacke Ram is tupping your White Ewe', he does not mean that the lovers are to be found, chalk in hand, at the blackboard of the Maths Faculty in the University of Venice. By the same token, we might regret how the honourable noun 'doctor', in spawning the verb 'to doctor', risks being contaminated with hints of falsification and adulteration.

Sometimes, moreover, words will, like boomerangs, turn back on themselves in mid-flight and, ungratefully and disloyally, injure the innocence of their origin. Thus: the man whose wife is adulterously tupped himself becomes a tup, the word (in a salt-in-wound kind of way) now coming to mean a cuckold, smearing the victim with the verbal overtones of the crime itself. Is general practice still a craft? Not if it implies we are crafty. A profession, then? Not if, as Ivan Illich insisted, to professionalise medicine is to conspire to disempower our patients. If thrown mud sticks, who would be a potter?

And it doesn't end there. You might also recall how, following my 'sheep' piece, I was chided by a correspondent for making play with his wife's maiden name, Tupp. He threatened to have me tupped (which, I learned to my relief, meant arrested, not sodomized) by the bogeys (meaning police, not nasal crusts). Luckily we never met face to face. Had we done so, I'd not have given tuppence for my chances in a fist-fight. (That's tuppence as in two old pennies, not, as you might have thought, the cost of hiring a ram on an overnight basis.)

Forgive me; I apostrophise. (That's apostrophise as in addressing you rhetorically and in brackets, not as in forming plural's like greengrocers's.) But something deadly serious underlies these admittedly enjoyable jugglings with words.

As I write, we are at war with Iraq, and the proposed new GMS contract has run aground on the rocks of the Carr-Hill formula. Words like 'moral' (as in moral high ground) or 'united' (as in United Nations), words like 'quality' (as in quality indicators) or 'opportunity' (as in earnings opportunity) are squirming to preserve any vestige of their original purity of meaning. What are we to make of it? Simply, inevitably, regrettably this; words, surreptitiously hi-jacked and ruthlessly wielded, are weapons of mass deception.

So let us be clear. In the context of our own unashamedly professional endeavours, and despite the obfuscations of our politicians, posturing is not the same as policy. Activity is not the same as action. Exhaustion is not the same as achievement. Protocols, guidelines and formulae are not the same as wisdom. And – as any dancing bear will tell you – new chains do not a new contract make.

6

Excuse me, doctor, I'm talking to you!

Considering how much of any reputation I've gained has sprung from my 1987 book *The inner consultation* (subtitled *how to develop an effective and intuitive consulting style*), I seem to have been pretty reticent on the subject of consulting skills ever since. In print, at any rate[1]. I suppose (i) I banged on about it as much as is decent in that book, and (ii) I've grown rather depressed at how much of a meal we seem to make of what ought, surely, to be a perfectly straightforward aspect of humane doctoring. Fundamentally — until we start trying to analyse, model and teach them — consulting skills are no different from the communication skills we all employ in ordinary social life when we're genuinely trying to understand or influence another person. When we want to sell a used car, for instance, or get off with someone at a party.

After all, what are we talking about? Nothing more complicated than:

- getting on the other person's wavelength
- paying attention to what they're saying
- reading between the lines
- planning the next move
- arranging to meet up again.

Every love-smitten teenager does all these without the slightest difficulty, and would laugh in your face if you reminded them, before they went out clubbing, to make sure they'd boned up on their communication skills.

So those of us who presume to teach young doctors how to be more effective in the way they talk with patients should be asking ourselves not, 'How can we give them a crash course in a foreign language?', but rather, 'How do we transpose the everyday ability to communicate into a professional setting?'

I guess that's the hard part — the 'professional setting'. One definition of a professional is someone who can do what they have to even when they don't feel like it. Anyone can be a good communicator in ideal circumstances; but doctors have to work at doing it on purpose, with sometimes unprepossessing patients, and when the purely medical aspects of the consultation are difficult enough.

---

[1] The 2nd edition of *The inner consultation* (2004) Radcliffe Publishing, contains an update on the present state of consulting skills and how they fit into the vocational training curriculum.

This chapter presents two pieces touching on different ways of developing a doctor's consulting style. The first is a review of the fourth book in a series arising from the Balint movement[2]. The other makes the point that patients remain our most effective teachers.

The doctor, the patient and the group[3]

It was P G Wodehouse who observed that the art of writing was the art of applying the seat of the trousers to the seat of the chair. The art of reading, it might be added, is the art of applying the point of the pen to the dotted line of the charge card slip. Books there will always be, because there will always be authors, and – fatwahs included – no known way of stopping them. An author, if anyone needs a definition, is someone convinced that the best person to learn from his or her experience is someone *else*. The latest book in the Balint canon has five authors.

The doctor, the patient and – wait for it! – *the group* is subtitled *Balint revisited*. Shouldn't that be *Balint re-re-visited*? There's the original *The D, his P and the illness*. Then there's the rather slimmer *Six minutes for the patient*, which described the flash[4]. Next came the slimmest and zappiest of all, *While I'm here, Doc*. Now we have *and the group*, weighing in at a noticeably heavier 162 pages. If these were successive human progeny we'd start wondering about diabetes in the mother, with an over-rich maternal metabolism producing an overgrown but paradoxically frail infant. There is, I have to say, a grain of truth in this rather flip analogy. I yield to no one in doffing my cap in homage to Michael Balint's bequest to British general practice, and maybe we shouldn't be counting, but I wonder whether the Balintian well isn't becoming just a bit – well – over-bucketed.

All of us who have had experience of what being in a Balint group can confer – the almost ecstatic realisation that what goes on inside the doctor is understandable, useful, usable and ultimately uplifting will appreciate the urge to share and to evangelise. The essence of the Balint approach is to take the patient's distress and pass it on, reflecting at every stage. The patient tells the doctor, and the doctor tells the group. So far, so good. But the next stage – the group tells the world – seems less essential. In these Chinese whispers, the purity of the message risks getting lost. For the Balint approach is primarily an experiential one. It requires real-life, real-time participation in seminars, week on week and year on year. Reading about it is not the same as experiencing. Balint books should be read as advertisements for the method, not short-cuts to it.

---

[2] Michael Balint was a Hungarian psychoanalyst who, settling in London in the 1950s, instigated a process (the 'Balint group') whereby practising GPs met regularly to discuss the psychodynamics of their interactions with patients. The Balint movement has had enormous influence on the development of the British understanding of the doctor-patient relationship, and continues to thrive. It represents what the patient had in mind when she said to her GP, 'Don't just *do* something – *sit there!*' The work of the original Balint group was written up as *The doctor, his patient and the illness* (1957) Pitman, London, and remains a classic to be recommended to all aspiring GPs.

[3] Balint E, Courtenay M et al. (1993) *The doctor, the patient and the group*. London, Routledge. Review excerpted from *Postgraduate Education for General Practice* (1993), **4**, 157–8.

[4] The 'flash' – a moment of insight when, the ground having been prepared by analysis of their previous relationship, patient or doctor suddenly understands the significance of puzzling symptoms or behaviour.

With that off my chest, there is much to commend in *The D, the P and the G*. Its self-appointed task is to examine what since the 1950s remains useful, what should be discarded, and what has been discovered. The book not so much fails in this mission as ignores it. Luckily. The Balint movement does not need a chairman's report. Instead, it translates into more contemporary language and contexts the experiences of a group of GPs whose sophistication is both admirable and well within the grasp of all of us, new contract or no new contract.

The core insight is summarized afresh as 'to take the (doctor's) observer-error seriously'. In a nice analogy to the laws of Newtonian physics, the doctor-patient relationship is reckoned to 'remain in a state of rest or uniform motion in a straight line, unless it is compelled by impressed forces to change that state'. What are these 'impressed forces', which may disturb the consultation or the relationship? They include novelty, the element of surprise, the accumulation of experience and the pain thereby engendered. In true Balint tradition, the participants' painful hacking of a path through the clinical undergrowth is documented *verbatim*. But in this book, even more than its predecessors, the quality of the written language is poetic and compelling, and it's a rattling good read.

Enid Balint[5], incidentally, writes in her introduction:

> 'It seems that general practitioners can feel inadequate because they are not specialists, but very few specialists feel inadequate because they are not general practitioners and therefore do not know how to work with patients who have no illness requiring specialist help.'

I'd rather thought that most course organisers and GP tutors spent much of their time trying to make their hospital colleagues realise precisely this inadequacy!

On consultation skills[6]

When I were a spotty lad – and I still have my 1963 bottle of crumbling tetracycline labelled 'The Tablets' to prove it – the general practice consultation was an altogether brisker and more straightforward affair. Make (or pretend to make) a diagnosis, prescribe or refer, ring the bell for the next patient. Sorted. (Ironic to think that then, when GPs had time for longer consultations, they didn't bother; whereas now, when we don't, we must.)

Readers of these pages will know that I'm not above a little hypocrisy, as long as it's sincere. So I confess to sometimes wondering whether we aren't in danger of elevating the consultation process to something rather more sophisticated than is good for it. As well as (and sometimes instead of) just being how someone's health problem gets fixed, the consultation has become a roller-coaster ride through a giddy terrain of extra tasks, goals and processes of which the patient is usually unaware. It's when we doctors get out our consultation models. It's our chance to dress up as an advocate or a freedom fighter, and see if we can get our heads round words like 'autonomy', 'empowerment', 'narrative' and 'transference'. It's when we play games like 'hit the target', and 'pass the protocol' and 'hunt the hidden agenda'.

---

[5] Michael Balint's wife, herself a psychoanalyst and Balint group leader for some years after her husband's death.
[6] *Behind the lines*, Back Pages, *Brit. J. Gen. Pract.*, November 2002.

It's actually not the consultation that's got complicated: despite all the flim-flam it still comes down to 'do as you would be done by'. But golly! – haven't we made an obstacle course out of learning how to do it. Books, models, checklists, courses, videos, role-plays. All this to try and make young doctors look experienced, and experienced ones behave as if they were idealistic young students again. But luckily, if we let them, the patients remain our ever-present and most effective teachers. Two case studies, both cross-my-heart true.

Old Henry

Henry, aged 72, has a swollen testicle. As he tells me about it, I know he thinks – and I think he knows I know he thinks – it's cancer. But the history's not right: and, when he's up on the couch, it looks to me like an epididymo-orchitis. Phew. Well, probably 'phew'. Time to manage uncertainty, remember safety-netting. 'I'm pretty sure it's just an infection …' I begin: ' … a urine sample … prescribe a course of … see you in a week.'

Phew, he's thinking, and his confidence starts to return. 'How've I got that then?' he asks. Damn. I reach into that cupboard in my mind where I keep the flannel. 'As we get older … the bladder … the prostate …' Henry knows I'm bluffing. 'Can you get it from sex?'

I'm well on to the back foot by now, and couldn't spot a minimal cue if it bit me on the knee.

''Cos if so,' he continues, 'it must have a bloody long incubation period.'

Young Giles

Giles, aged eight, has a skin tag on the side of his nose, and his mother says he wants it removed. Hmm, I think patient-centredly, painful place to put local anaesthetic in; and I say as much. 'Oh,' says his mum, expressing her Ideas-Concerns-and-Expectations as to the manner born, 'I thought you'd just tie a bit of cotton round it.' 'Okay,' says I, grateful for the chance to Incorporate Her Health Beliefs. So Giles climbs up on the couch while I prepare a loose knot of black Sylko and advance on my target. Ethical dilemma: shall I tell him it will hurt for a moment? If I do, he'll flinch and I'll miss with the noose and it'll all … So I think 'stuff informed consent' and just do it. I lasso the skin tag, give a quick yank, and snip off the loose ends. Sorted.

Well, Giles is eight, which is nearly grown up, so although I've brought tears to his eyes he manages not to yelp. And they both get up to leave. 'Come back,' says his mother, 'what do you say to the doctor?' And Giles, aged eight, his hand already on the door handle, looks me in the eye and says in a shaky treble, 'You bastard.'

Maybe some complexities are best left undeconstructed, some pretty jigsaws left intact and not pulled apart into pieces for clumsy fingers to fiddle with. Best just enjoyed. I reckon we need fewer educational paradigms, and more teachers like Giles and Henry.

7

'Values authentic and pure?'[1]

In one camp there are authors who spend years – lifetimes, often amassing experience and 'memos to self' until, opinionated to bursting point, they can't *not* write it all down. For them, the virgin page is like a bed-pan brought in the nick of time. And in the other camp are others – jaundiced hacks for the most part, on a 'so much a thousand words' contract – to whom that same virgin page is as irresistible as a graffiti-free wall to a kid with a spray can. Me? I've a foot in both; camps, that is.

When all you have is a hammer, everything looks like a nail. And so to a writer with a deadline, an awful lot of one-liners look like promising kick-starts to a piece of brilliant prose. Call up a new blank document on the word processor, type in a *bon mot* from your little black notebook, and then free-wheel on your powers of association and lateral thinking. 'Politics is the art of pulling wool over blind eyes', you write (or something equally sententious) – and see where the notion takes you. (Actually, that's quite good; I must write it up somewhere.)

On the other hand, it's been my experience that whatever thoughts bubble up after tossing a random pebble into the depths of the authorial psyche seem to be things you'd actually always known, but had hitherto neglected to articulate until the blank page compelled you.

Or, to put it succinctly but unoriginally, I'm one of those people who doesn't know what they think until they see what they say.

Looking back through the *Behind the lines* columns I wrote monthly for two years, I notice that many of them were prompted by observations which, if not entirely random, were at least not pre-planned. The blue-bottomed sheep of Dumfries, for example, or the maraudings of Harold Shipman. The first piece in this section, 'On poetry', is in this category. Late in 2002 the new contract for GPs was being mooted, threatening, as it then seemed, through enticement and bribery to exchange clinical freedom for obedience. It was easy at the time to feel nostalgic for the institutions and working methods of my professional youth, and a chance encounter in the *Guardian* of a line of T E Hulme pressed this button. Nostalgia is a difficult thing to argue logically for, but – and I know it's a cop-out – the persuasive power of a decent metaphor can be more than a match for logic.

---

[1] 'The authentic and pure values – truth, beauty, and goodness – in the activity of a human being are the result of one and the same act, a certain application of the full attention to the object.'
Simone Weil (1909–1943): *La pesanteur et la grâce* (1948)

In other words (I hope), be true to your own reality, and what you come up with will be true.

In the haunting words of Gaston Bachelard[2], 'The image has touched the depths before it stirs the surface.'

The other pieces in this chapter are also taken from the *Back pages*. 'On caring' was written immediately after learning I had been elected President of the RCGP. It was odd, and probably a panic reaction — but the prospect of high office seemed to jolt me into trying to get clear in my own mind just what I thought mattered about the general practice way of doctoring. One core principle of general practice — and I hope history won't show this too to have been just nostalgia — is that caring is a verb. 'Care' is something that we doctors *do*, not a commodity we arrange the delivery of.

On the evidence of the next few pieces, it seems I also think that something more than fine words is needed to butter the parsnips of the new contract (for the parsnip story, *see* page 39); that general practice is a performance art; that vocation might be a myth but I still want to believe in it. The piece 'On professionalism' was my last *Behind the lines* column. I recognised that, as College President, it behoved me to be more circumspect about sounding off in public. Since then (and in the wake of the Shipman disaster), it has become even more urgent to re-establish that being a professional is a matter of pride and some guarantee of responsibility. We can start by being clear and explicit about our own professional values. But — given that as professionals we are in a three-way reciprocal relationship with the public and the policy-makers — it will help if the said public and policy-makers can in turn be equally clear and explicit about theirs[3].

On poetry[4]

With the possible exception of Henry 'Naming of parts' Reed[5], I don't really do poetry. When I am informed by the late Lord Tennyson that ' "Tirra lirra" by the river Sang Sir Lancelot', none of the rejoinders which spring to my lips reflect well on either knight or poet, nor indeed on my own Plebeian self. I relate more to Nigel 'the curse of St Custards' Molesworth, who, compelled to recite aloud, records the ensuing artistic treat thus[6]:

---

[2] Gaston Bachelard (1884–1962). French scientist, philosopher and poet. Quotation from the introduction to his *The poetics of space* (English translation 1969) Beacon Press, Boston.

[3] I'm glad to report that, even as I write, this agenda is being picked up by influential colleagues. Carol Black, President of the Royal College of Physicians and contributor of the Foreword to this book, is setting up a working party on 'defining and maintaining medical professionalism', chaired by Baroness Cumberledge and of which I am a member.

[4] *Behind the lines*, Back Pages, *Brit. J. Gen. Pract.*, January 2003.

[5] Henry Reed (1914–1986). Second World War poet, broadcaster and playwright. His best-known poem, *Naming of parts*, a parody on army basic training, cuts between the brutish voice of the instructor and the private musings of a recruit:

> This is the lower sling swivel. And this
> Is the upper sling swivel, whose use you will see,
> When you are given your slings. And this is the piling swivel,
> Which in your case you have not got. The branches
> Hold in the gardens their silent, eloquent gestures,
> Which in our case we have not got.

[6] Willans G and Searle R (1984) *The compleet Molesworth: how to be topp in English*. Pavilion Books, London.

SIR THE BURIAL SIR OF SIR JOHN MOORE SIR AT CORUNNA SIR
(A titter from 2B they are wet and i will tuough them up after.)
Notadrumwasheardnotafuneralnote
shut up peason larffing
As his corse
As his corse
what is a corse sir? Gosh is it
to the rampart we carried
(whisper you did not kno your voice was so lovely)
Not a soldier discharged his farewell shot.
PING!
Shut up peason i know sir he's blowing peas at me
Oer the grave where our hero we buried.

But now and again the occasional line does press some button, does jab one in the fleshy parts, does cause to flash before the mind's eye some truth which, albeit less than clearly discerned, nevertheless cries undeniably for expression. I chanced recently upon this, from T E Hulme's *'Images'*[7]

Old houses were scaffolding once and workmen whistling.

The wretched thing's persistent, won't get out of my head. 'Old houses were scaffolding once and workmen whistling': there's a medical metaphor in there somewhere, I can smell it. And while I don't do poetry, I do do metaphor – which is odd, because they're essentially the same thing. To a prose-monger like me, metaphor is truth with wings, and poetry just metaphor in fancy dress. Anyway, at risk of showing myself up for the unreconstructed fuddy-duddy which at heart I probably am (and which we are all destined to become), I'm driven to try and unpack Hulme's metaphor.

Is he simply saying, 'What's now old was once new'? I guess not; a poet couldn't be that blindingly obvious. 'Even the most enduring of our institutions emerged from the mud and confusion of a building site.'? That perhaps comes closer. Then again – since I'm from a generation to whom age in a house suggests character and craftsmanship rather than dry rot and noisy plumbing – Hulme could be reminding us that 'what now looks out of date and irrelevant was once created with skill and dedication, and should be respected for it'. Is the poet warning the young not to belittle their heritage? Or the old not to laud it over the new kids on the block, nor hold their inexperience against them? Yes. And no. That's poetry for you. Ambiguous.

I look around the urban skyline of my own professional habitat. Backlit by a setting sun are silhouetted some of the structures that have given my working life a sense of place and purpose. Vocational training, which is intended to give young GPs the time – and, more importantly, the permission and the freedom – to explore their own curiosity. The Balint movement, and all the creative interest in the doctor-patient relationship and the consultation process that flowed from it. All the local variations on one fundamental architectural design, that places the resources of the individual doctor at the service of the needs of the individual

---

[7] Thomas Ernest Hulme (1883–1917). Staffordshire-born poet of the First World War, killed in action on the Western Front.

patient. Old buildings these may be; but I've in my turn put up a few scaffolding poles and done a fair bit of whistling, and I'm fond of them. So while I understand that new ways of doing medicine need new homes and premises, I do wish 'development' wasn't so often a euphemism for demolition.

The JCBs and ball-hammers are at work on the brown-field building site that is to become the new general practice. And what does the architect's model promise? A patchwork estate, some of it mock Georgian, the rest a mix of the jerry-built and the trompe-l'oeil. And who is to live in Newtown-Blair? A dwindling generation of cash-strapped, target-driven, protocol-worshipping, initiative-purged young doctors, too busy to notice where they're living and too stressed to care much.

Gosh. Maybe there's something in this poetry malarkey after all. I feel a New Year's Resolution coming on: look more carefully for the poetical in practice. I might even attempt the odd line of my own. In fact, I'll start right now by reworking Hulme.

New houses are scaffolding still and builders bickering.

On caring[8]

Standing for election, like knowing one is to be hanged in a fortnight, concentrates the mind wonderfully. The nomination form for the 2003–2006 RCGP Presidency called for a manifesto, a summary of one's ambitions for the College, in not more than 100 words. Given that I've taken nearly 15 000 words so far in my *Behind the lines* pieces sounding off about what I think is good and bad about general practice, the College and the political context in which we live, breathe and have our struggling, a mere hundred should have been easy. But actually it wasn't. 'Cut the crap,' the form seemed to be saying. 'Ditch the funny stuff. Tell us what you *really* believe.'

So I tried; and rediscovered that saying what you're *for* is harder than saying what you're *against*. And telling it straight is harder than telling it funny. 'The President's job is to give a lead on values,' I wrote, after much agonizing. 'Mine are uncompromisingly those of the consulting room, where individual doctors bring knowledge, resources, insight, experience and commitment to the service of individual patients. The challenge for the College and the NHS is to preserve consulting-room values in the face of short-term political expedients and the over-regulation of professional judgement.'

Yesterday I learned the result of the ballot. I am to be your next President, succeeding Dame Lesley Southgate, who has achieved great things as a personal doctor, an academic, and an arbiter of high-quality practice. Two four-letter words about sum up my immediate reaction, the second being, 'Gulp!' Huge is the honour, and huge the responsibility. And huge are the opportunities to secure for personal doctoring the recognition it deserves as the embodiment of all that is good, and sound, and worthy, and thoughtful, and cost-effective in delivering care to the nation's unwell – who are, after all, the friends and neighbours and relations of us all.

Then today I remembered that I need to get my copy for the July *Back Pages* in to Alec the Editor. And dammit – the urge to be up front about what I believe is

---

[8] *Behind the lines*, Back Pages, *Brit. J. Gen. Pract.*, July 2003.

still with me. But how to do it? Nothing more undermines the sense of humour than the prospect of having to put one's performance where one's mouth is. And (as any columnist will tell you) principles that cannot be expressed are hardly worth having. I think it all hinges on this word 'care'.

What a complex and two-faced word 'care' has become. In Orwell's *Nineteen Eighty-Four* the Ministry of Love was in fact the agency for imposing repression. Similarly, care – at least when the word is bandied around by those state agencies charged with lowering voters' expectations – is all too often the smiling face of indifference. In disgracefully many official documents, bunging the word 'care' into titles and text is calculated to press a positive response button, much as claiming to have hit your head is the way to fast-track your sprained ankle through A & E, or professing green sputum guarantees you antibiotics for a cold.

Of *course* patients deserve to receive good, focused, evidence-informed clinical care – the better the better. If quality agendas and targets and new contracts will achieve this, more strength to their bony little elbows. But I think patients want to be more than the recipients of formalised care bestowed upon them by a state machine desperate to be perceived as competent: I think they want to be cared *for*. More importantly (and least quantifiably), patients want to be cared *about* – cared about by the doctors who care for them. There is a risk in the latest attempts to redefine good practice that pursuit of the abstract noun 'care' could come to substitute for the active verb 'to care'. The equating of caring with care could invalidate the balance sheet where the value of general practice is determined.

In Peter Shaffer's 1973 play *Equus*, there's a moment in which Martin Dysart, a child psychiatrist close to burnout, is confiding in his magistrate friend, Hesther. 'Of course,' she says ironically, 'I feel totally fit to be a magistrate all the time.' And he replies, 'No, you don't – but then that's you feeling unworthy to fill a job. I feel the job is unworthy to fill *me*.' How dangerous it would be if the 'Dysart doubt' were to become widespread in general practice. What a tragedy, if a rising generation of GPs were to find that professional life in a target-driven culture which sets too high a premium on slavish delivery of formulaic care proved insufficiently worthy of their intelligence and devotion.

For everyone's sake, primary care, and our College in particular, must continue to champion the primacy of caring. *Cum scientia calculatio?*[9] I don't think so.

On parsnips[10]

The RCGP has its motto – '*Cum scientia caritas*'. And it has its heraldic crest – an arrangement of assorted fauna, pressed flowers and bric-a-brac. What it has hitherto lacked is a signature dish. Michel Bras has his *gargouillou de jeunes légumes*, Heston Blumenthal (it wouldn't surprise me) his *raviolo of marshmallow on an oyster coulis*. True, the College does a very decent full English breakfast, healthily defiant of any guideline ever published. But can we match our sister Royal College of Surgeons' *tripes à la chirurgique*, the Paediatricians' *oeuf à la coque avec ses soldats*, or the spotted dick reputedly so popular with our Obs and Gynae colleagues?

---

[9] The motto of the Royal College of General Practitioners is, '*Cum scientia caritas*' – 'compassion with knowledge'.

[10] *Behind the lines*, Back Pages, *Brit. J. Gen. Pract.*, September 2003.

I think every institution worth its salt should make a unique contribution to world gastronomy. So, on behalf of our own College (and, as ever, in search of a half-decent metaphor), I propose *panais au beurre* – buttered parsnips. Let me explain.

The profession has accepted the new contract by a majority that will be interpreted by its supporters as a resounding 'yes', and by dissenters as a heavily qualified 'yes but'. It would be hard, indeed churlish, to argue against the principle of rewarding GPs in proportion to our performance in delivering consistent and high-quality clinical care. Moreover, we should know by now that the present Government, like every other six-year-old, wants to hear the loudest possible bang for its buck.

But there remain plenty among us who fear that, in too headlong a pursuit of performance markers many of which are mere eye-candy or window-dressing, some of the precious, delicate and subtle characteristics of good patient-centred doctoring might get trampled underfoot. Skills that presently give substance to the speciality of generalism are in danger of atrophying until they are no more than the fine words which proverbially butter no parsnips.

The first Elizabethan age saw the geographical world explored and its diversity harvested. Foods once exotic – tomatoes, potatoes – were brought back from remote lands and quickly adopted as staples. In the new Elizabethan age, it is the world of ideas which has been similarly opened up, not least by general practice. We GPs have a long tradition of navigating successfully beyond our own territorial waters. We have made reckless but profitable raids into the home-lands of psychiatrists, psychologists, family therapists, social workers, educationists, accountants, novelists, mystics, priests – and have brought back a booty of techniques and philosophies to enrich our patient care. Look along your bookshelves and see the names of the Walter Raleighs and Vasco da Gamas of our own time: Pickles, Balint, Byrne, Horder, Widgery, Pendleton, Willis, Heath ...

Probably the key quality possessed by explorers in every domain is curiosity – a passion to know why and how things are as they are, and whether they couldn't be better. If we try to carry this attitude into the more mundane world of the new contract we have a difficult balancing act to bring off. We have to be at once cooperative and critical, constructive and curious, challenged and challenging.

But if anybody can be good at reconciling so many tensions, it ought to be us. GPs thrive on the kind of fuzzy thinking that can on the one hand do *this* while on the other not forgetting *that*. The parsnips of good clinical governance need to be dressed with the butter of curiosity. But the case for preserving curiosity – for flair, for individuality, for creativity, for (let's face it) style – is going to need sustained advocacy. I think that's one thing the College should lead on. If CAMRA can do it for beer, I'm sure the RCGP can be an effective focus in a Campaign for Real General Practice. The resources of a national College like ours can, I suspect, be put to no better use than encouraging and promulgating original thought within our discipline – and seeing that it trickles out past Princes Gate[11], past Richmond House[12], past Downing Street and Parliament Square, and into every consulting room in the land.

---

[11] 14 Princes Gate, London SW7 1PU is the address of the RCGP.
[12] The Whitehall headquarters of the Department of Health.

In his piece on the new contract in last month's *Back Pages* David Hannay lamented 'the end of general practice as we know it'. To the extent that the old contract camouflaged the odd pocket of sloppy or shoddy practice, or the occasional self-indulgent or self-deluding doctor, we should not mourn its passing. But for the new one to be worthy of support and respect, it must not stop at deterring the worst of us: it must encourage the best in us.

It should be to the College that colleagues, patients, politicians and administrators look in order to know what is 'the best in us'. It is up to us to be worthy of that expectation. Or, if you like, to be the butter on the parsnips.

On performance[13]

If it's still on when you read this, and if you possibly can, catch Tom Stoppard's *Jumpers* at the National Theatre. This farce, which I saw premiered in 1972 – oh God!, the year I started vocational training – this ever-fresh farce brings into unlikely collision the disparate worlds of philosophy and acrobatics.

George our crumpled hero, stunningly played by becardiganed Simon Russell Beale, is that general practitioner of the academic world, the Professor of Moral Philosophy. He is flagrantly cuckolded by the smooth-talking consultant-resembling Archie – Vice Chancellor, psychiatrist and amateur acrobat. Another member of the acrobatic squad has been inadvertently shot by George's wife, Dotty. Complications, as they say, set in.

I love word-play, and Stoppard's delicious linguistic pyrotechnics have me in Heaven. For example: George, an amateur archer, soliloquising on Zeno's paradox, convinces himself that 'though an arrow is always approaching its target, it never quite gets there, and Saint Sebastian died of fright.' Laugh? Till the tears ran down my leg.

Why am I telling you this? Several weeks have gone by since I saw the play, and like all good art it's left something behind inside me, niggling away. It's hard to put into words; bear with me.

Many GPs find their work engenders a form of spiritual fidgeting, a reaching-out for deeper meaning, an inclination to squeeze a little significance out of life's spitefulnesses. As doctors, we are valued for the empathic way we can come alongside individual people in their individual extremity, and simultaneously for our role as the wise and detached professional. It comforts patients to think we can see the big picture while they carry on suffering the small ones. For a doctor to view patients' predicaments as so many wrinkles in the fabric of the universe is not callous or dismissive. It helps; for if we can take them in our stride, then – by proxy – so can they.

In a word, the job makes philosophers of us, philosophers of the Stoic persuasion. Since we too are mortal and made of wrinkles, it takes a lot of practice to look uncrumpled, to act unfazed. And there is a sense, too, in which we must be acrobats. Good doctoring calls for balance, timing, cooperation and agility – if not of the body, at least of the intellect. The dropped catch, the fatal plummet is only a fumble away.

---

[13] *Behind the lines*, Back Pages, *Brit. J. Gen. Pract.*, October 2003.

I think the niggling heresy with which Stoppard has infected me is the wish to recognise general practice as a performance art. I don't mean simply in the 'All the world's a stage' sense, which holds people, ourselves included, to be no more than the portfolio of roles in their repertoire. Anthony Rooley, in a book on performance[14], takes the Shakespearean view, seeing all our actions, every interplay of relationships and pursuits of all kinds as 'performance'. 'At times,' he acknowledges, 'it seems as though such a view may take all spontaneity out of everything, only for us to discover that potentially it leads to yet greater freedom.' Rooley suggests that 'if we play our roles with ease, unselfconsciously, with love and care, then through our play we may blossom, and those around us too.'

If we buy into the idea of 'general practice as performance', and its corollary that GPs are actors, we must also accept the problems that go with it. Not least is the fundamental irony every actor faces — if he[15] is to move the audience, he must himself remain unmoved and in command of his performance. This is an old chestnut. The 18th century French man of letters Denis Diderot argued[16] that great actors must possess judgement and penetration without 'sensibility' — i.e., without actually experiencing the emotions they are portraying as characters on the stage. For to do so would be to lose the ability to lift the audience/patient to yet greater insights. Diderot asked how the actor is to catch just the point at which he must stop being himself and become the practitioner of a contrived and well-rehearsed skill. He couldn't answer his own question; but then, he'd not had the benefit of being in a Balint group.

That great theatre takes place, albeit unwitnessed, in the consulting room few will deny. Occasionally Shakespearean in its import, it is more often Ibsen, or else Alan Ayckbourn. No stage or TV drama has quite captured the cameo subtleties of the two-handers played out between GP and patient every ten minutes. Yet the consultation provides a ritual which (to quote Rooley again) 'in the moment of performance has relevance for our entire lives. The experience of performance contains such powerful things: heightened states of awareness, moments of incredible clarity, profound admiration and respect.'

Gosh. Do we hear applause? I wish.

On vocation[17]

At school I was never any good at sport. On the rare occasions when my mother, in a cruel access of Puritanism, withheld the usual 'off games' note, and the last few shivering ball-bunglers were being allocated to the Skins or the Jerseys for the weekly kick-around, it was always, 'Sir, do we *have* to have Neighbour? We had him *last* time.'

Not that it didn't hurt. So imagine how hopefully my ears pricked up when our GP Dr Heap, shown the itchy mankiness between my toes, diagnosed athlete's foot. Athlete's?, I thought: Well, it's a start. But it was not to be; after only a few

---

[14] Rooley A (1990) *Performance: revealing the Orpheus within*. Element Books, Longmead.
[15] Sorry about the sexist pronouns. When the English language cracks it, let me know.
[16] Diderot D (1713–1784) *Paradoxe sur le comédien (The paradox of acting)*: written in 1773, published in 1830.
[17] *Behind the lines*, Back Pages, *Brit. J. Gen. Pract.*, November 2003.

applications of his tincture of gentian violet, the fungus, and with it any dream of sporting prowess, was expunged.

Now there's magic for you — a man who can look at your foot and read your soul, paint the one bright purple and, with the hot poultice of truth, surreptitiously cast out foolish imaginings from the other. I remember wanting to do things like that.

In the sensible days when medical students were selected by interview, Tutors for Admission were wont to divide candidates into two groups — those who claimed their vocation to become doctors stemmed from reading *Middlemarch*, and the rest. This latter, smaller, set included an implausible few who asserted, road-to-Damascus-style, that it came to them in a blinding flash that their mission in life was to Heal The Sick. Rather more conceded that, having got good grades in science A-levels, it was, like, kind of, inevitable. A few cocky souls boasted that since everybody, or nobody, in their family was a doctor, their destiny was to conform to, or break, the mould. A brave but honest rump, asked why they wanted to be doctors and biting back an unimpressive 'Dunno', struggled to express with acceptable eloquence the simple fact that they hadn't a clue whence sprang their motivation, and that, with respect, the question was a silly one.

I'd have been one of the 'dunno's. Personally, I've always been sceptical that so priggishly evangelical a doctor as George Eliot's Tertius Lydgate could inspire anyone to anything other than the urge to throttle him. (So marrying the mayor's socially ambitious daughter proved his ruin? Serve him right, I say: if he'd spent less time puffing the virtues of scientific progress and more on buffing up his communication skills, he'd have been a happier man.) And I've never had a Damascus-road experience, not unless you count the realisation that golf is a silly game. What's more, no one in my family was medical; but I don't recall ever holding that against them, nor feeling any great weight of expectation on my youthful shoulders. I just know I never wanted to do anything else: not for long, anyway. But where does vocation come from?

And indeed, what *is* vocation? To a person untouched by it, I guess to have a vocation seems like something noble, something to be envied, something that saves a whole bunch of trouble at the Careers Convention. From the inside, though, isn't it more like this: a sense that one's destiny is in the unseen but reliable hands of some inevitability that whispers life's destination in your ear even as you get under way? The voice that whispers is often indistinct, though in my own case it was Dr Heap's if it was anybody's.

Even so, I can't quite accept that something as banal as the athlete's foot incident was enough reason to embark on a career which, however much I've enjoyed it in hindsight, was in its early stages often distasteful, exhausting, and seemingly disconnected from the furtherance of human well-being.

I don't know — I really don't know — whether there is such a thing as vocation. It's an attractive badge for one's professional motives, and can disguise (if disguise is called for) a host of less laudable needs: status, power, money, security, atonement, vicarious intimacy. But one can feel driven without there necessarily being a driver. Moreover, it's the car's engine that propels it, not the go-faster stripes emblazoned *post hoc* on its sides. Oh! the unanswered questions. Is vocation after all a mythical beast, like Nessie or the Phoenix? Extinct like the dodo, or, like the panda, cuddly but endangered? A parasite like mistletoe, nourished only by the living sap of sturdier rationales? A dream, a false memory, a fictitious invention of the questioned mind?

Whatever. It is certain that something sometimes happens – fortunately – to impel the unsuspecting young towards this most marvellous of jobs. And I wish we knew how to spot it, foster it, select for it. The Scottish educationist A S Neill once pondered, 'If we have to have an exam at 11, let us make it one for humour, sincerity, imagination, character – and where is the examiner who could test such qualities?' And I reply, 'I don't know, but I hope there's one on every medical school selection panel.'

On professionalism[18]

'Start by grabbing the reader's attention' is the gist of Lesson One on most creative writing courses. OK then. Professional is the new gay.

Or rather, 'professional' is the new 'gay'. Note the quotation marks. The word 'professional' is currently experiencing the same dizzy shifts in connotation latterly undergone by the word 'gay'. In the 1960s, the 'brightly coloured' or 'carefree' meanings of 'gay' were supplanted by the 'homosexual' one, so that (as the *New Oxford Dictionary* puts it) 'the word cannot readily be used unselfconsciously in these older senses without arousing a sense of *double entendre*'.

Time was, being a professional was a matter of pride and a badge of integrity. Joining a profession entailed mastering a large corpus of knowledge – knowledge vital to the well-being of the ordinary individual, but more complex and extensive than every individual could hope to acquire. Professional training was long and preferably arduous, undertaken within a tradition of self-imposed discipline, of responsibility willingly accepted and of service willingly given. 'A professional is a man who can do his job when he doesn't feel like it. An amateur is a man who can't do his job even when he does feel like it.'[19] And in exchange for hard work and sacrifice, the professional deserved appreciation and generous reward.

But – for societies as much as for individuals – gratitude is a difficult thing to sustain without its turning to resentment. The medical profession in particular – dealing, sometimes disdainfully, with people's messier misfortunes – was bound sooner or later to attract criticism of the who-do-they-think-they-are variety. One notorious example was Ivan Illich's 1975 polemic *Medical nemesis*, beginning 'The medical establishment has become a major threat to health', (by causing more pathology – physical, spiritual and social – through its activities than ever it relieves)[20]. Illich is in the tradition of Bernard Shaw's well-known 'All professions are conspiracies against the laity'[21], (though we might smile wryly at the ambivalence that led Shaw later to write, in his preface to *Misalliance*, 'Optimistic lies have such immense therapeutic value that a doctor who cannot tell them convincingly has mistaken his profession'). And Ogden Nash's needle goes straight to the point of maximum tenderness: 'Professional men, they have no cares; Whatever happens, they get theirs.'[22]

Unfortunately the snipers are still out there, some of them in commanding vantage points. Julian Le Grand, Professor of Social Policy at the London School of

---

[18] *Behind the lines*, Back Pages, *Brit. J. Gen. Pract.*, December 2003.
[19] James Agate (1877–1947). British drama critic and novelist.
[20] Illich I (1975) *Medical nemesis: the expropriation of health*. Calder & Boyars, London.
[21] *The doctor's dilemma* (1911).
[22] *I yield to my learned brother* (1935).

Economics and currently on secondment to 10 Downing Street's policy unit, has recently published a book whose innocuous title, *Motivation, agency and public policy*, camouflages a powerful blunderbuss aimed at the professional heart[23]. You can just see its muzzle peeping out from the subtitle – *of knights & knaves, pawns & queens*. His thesis is that the motivation of professionals is more complicated than either pure altruism or pure self-interest, that patients are neither all-passive nor all-powerful, and that healthcare policy should be designed with these realities in mind.

So far, so true: thank you for noticing. But it's all too predictable what would happen when the journalists got hold of it. Beneath a headline proclaiming 'Public workers are "knaves", says Blair aide', The *Independent on Sunday* of 12th October said, 'Doctors ... who resist the Government's plans for reform are "knaves" motivated by plain self-interest.' Concerns that reform might pose a threat to the spirit of caring are 'likely to take the form of arrogant, insensitive, uncaring, overweening behaviour, even from professionals.'[24]

Grrrr. Professor Le Grand's powerful warning against the dangers of oversimplification may well itself have been oversimplified. But I'm too cross to enjoy the irony. It's almost irresistible to wonder, pot-and-kettle-like, whether Downing Street policy advisors are uniquely devoid of self-interest. Likewise to ask, sauce-for-goose-and-gander-like, whether – if professionalism means genuine accountability, job-specific training and willingness to subject one's motivation to unflinching scrutiny – we might not be better served by a Parliament of professionalised decision-makers.

But this sloganeering, point-scoring and name-calling doesn't help; it really, really does not help. Well, only if it succeeds in clearing the ground for the growth of mutual respect. We could start by trying to reclaim some dignity for the word 'professional', just as 'gay' has reclaimed a new dignity from the opprobrium of the recent past. How? By constant explanation. By constant advocacy. By the constant demonstration of good professionalism in action. And by the constant expectation that professionalism on the part of doctors will be reciprocated by those with whom we cooperate in the pursuit of an NHS to be proud of.

---

[23] Le Grand J (2003) *Motivation, agency and public policy*. Oxford University Press, Oxford. In May 2004 Professor Le Grand succeeded Simon Stevens as the Prime Minister's chief health advisor.
[24] Andy McSmith, Political Editor. *Independent on Sunday*, 12 Oct. 2003, p. 12.

8

A polished razor keen[1]

The Roman Juvenal (c. 55–127 AD) was the best and bravest of satirists. Best because he confined his barbs to the two most deserving targets – civic corruption, and the follies and brutalities of mankind. Bravest because he began his career as a literary sniper under one of Rome's most corrupt and brutal regimes, that of the much-feared emperor Domitian. Asked why he wrote satire, Juvenal (anticipating, perhaps, Mallory's 'Because it's there' reason for tackling Everest) quipped, 'Difficile est saturam non scribere': 'It's hard *not* to.' Twenty centuries later, looking around at the sleaze and silliness that still infects our public life and contaminates our decision-making processes, one knows what he means. Given, though, that twenty centuries later nothing much has changed, the satirist of today might equally wonder 'why bother?'

In this chapter are some far-from-brave attempts to poke a little well-merited fun at three of my own sources of irritation, albeit on a much more vernacular scale. First up is a piece lampooning the pandemic of mission statements which seems to have overtaken the medical and political establishments. Then comes an attempt to resolve an increasingly common source of confusion in the world of committees, the 'Pooh-Bah phenomenon', when multiple and sometimes conflicting vested interests are represented by a single individual who tries to wear too many hats at the same time, after the manner of the Lord High Everything Else in *The Mikado*. Finally (and I shall quite understand if the reader who wishes the book on the psychometrics of the MRCGP examination to remain closed prefers to skip this bit), a protest at the culture of assessment, and in particular its over-reliance on statistical analysis. This last piece, 'The Excalibur coefficient', is written as by my invented persona, the Radcliffe Armchair Professor of Clinical Philosophy.

On bititulism[2]

When did you last see a book with a proper title? OK, let's narrow it down a bit – a medical book with a simple crisp one-liner on the cover, in the tradition of William Harvey's classic *Exercitatio anatomica de motu cordis et sanguinis in animalibus*. One searches in vain for *Harry Potter and the Charnley hip prosthesis*, or *Everything you needed to know about Class II National Insurance contributions but were afraid to ask*.

---

[1] 'Satire should, like a polished razor keen,
  Wound with a touch that's scarcely felt or seen.'
                                        Lady Mary Worley Montagu (1689–1762)

[2] *Behind the lines*, Back Pages, *Brit. J. Gen. Pract.*, July 2002.

Nowadays every book seems to be bititular: it has two titles. The main one is short and (in the publishers' eyes at least) catchy, and Each Word Has An Initial Capital. Then there's a colon. Then, post-colonically, you get the subtitle, in lower case and considerably longer. Were modesty not to forbid, I could cite *The Inner Consultation: how to develop an effective and intuitive consulting style*. Even as I write, the *BMJ* carries a review of John Bunker's *Medicine Matters After All: measuring the benefits of medical care, a healthy lifestyle, and a just social environment*.

What's going on here? Is this bititulism a form of inverted familiarity, the opposite of 'My name's the Honourable Hector Arbuthnot-Smythe, but you can call me Snubby'? Maybe it's a sign of affluence — the two-car family preferring two-title books. Or a reflection of the tabloid/broadsheet split in our mass media — *Gotcha!: 368 feared lost as General Belgrano is sunk*.

This 'Grab 'em by the nose then lead 'em where you will' technique is the stock-in-trade of professional manipulators like hypnotists and advertising executives. So when politicians start doing it we should get nervous. Bititulism is now ubiquitous in the committee rooms of power. Remember the gloved fist of *Developing NHS Purchasing & GP Fundholding: towards a primary care-led NHS*, or the wittily-named *A Short Cut To Better Services: day surgery in England and Wales*? The latest example is the motherhood-and-apple-pie of *The NHS Plan: a plan for investment, a plan for reform*. Do you spot the theme? *Political Bititulism: a sound-bite and a follow-up platitude*.

You'd think we'd have learned by now; the point of such rhetorical tricks is to obfuscate with spurious sincerity. Two-part inventions like these are intended to soften us up so that, bleary-eyed with The Vision Thing, we don't notice the quicksand into which we are being enticed. *Two-Part Titles: a strategy for securing mindless acquiescence*.

Worse, bititulism has spawned an epidemic of banality in the form of a proliferation of cringe-making mission statements that so disfigure the thinking (or at least the letterheads) of our national institutions. You know the sort of thing: *Council Finance Office: balancing books for a better Bogthorpe*, or *The National Consortium of Double Glazing Salespersons: serving you right*. Closer to home we have the GMC, now *Protecting patients, guiding doctors*. Even the RCGP, no longer content with *Cum scientia caritas*, has dredged up *Promoting excellence in family medicine*. At least with the Latin, you knew what it meant.

I think somewhere there must be either a committee or a small plastic gizmo whose function is to generate this rubbish. It's easy enough — you start with an aspirational phrase such as 'towards' or 'striving for'. Follow it with some desirable-sounding and politically correct abstraction — fairness, perhaps, or service — and round it off with a phrase suggesting universality, e.g. 'in general practice' or 'for the new millennium'. If you can get three alliterative words into this bit, so much the better. The result is a slogan implying that we, like the Soviet comrades of old, are drones with fixed dilated grins marching in step behind the dictator's tawdry flag. *Creating Mission Statements: jingoistic gibberish for jugginses*.

Fun though it may be to laugh at the more outlandish examples of bititulism, or to think up one's own — *The Royal College of Midwives: pushing for progress in parturition*? — I have a serious purpose in sending it up. Two purposes, actually.

First, there is a danger that, by taking mission-statementism seriously, we fail to recognise the extreme of self-parody into which we may fall. By reducing a genuinely noble ambition to a silly slogan we risk (baby and bath-water-wise) allowing ourselves to abandon it. The mission statement cheapens the mission. The big pictures that ought to concern us – the well-being of individuals and the health of the nation – are too complex to be reduced to small-minded catch phrases.

Secondly, we should not shrink from denouncing the prevailing culture of oversimplification, nor from questioning the motives of our political masters who would have us subscribe to it. Whenever we see a two-part heading to a political initiative we should publicly and vociferously add a third – its real subtext. *The NHS plan: a plan for investment, a plan for reform.* In other words, *Doctors, do as the Government tells you, or go hungry. The RCGP: promoting excellence in family medicine – against all the odds.*

On the wearing of hats[3]

Certain convolutions of the probate laws, regrettably protracted, have recently delivered into my possession the literary effects of my great-great-aunt, the Victorian bluestocking and self-styled 'Doctor of Etiquette' Miss Laetitia Neighbour, formerly of Downapeg Mansions, London W1.

My late relative suffered for most of her fertile years from an unrequited passion for a succession of denizens of Harley Street, each of whom in turn eschewed her suggestion of matrimonial alliance in favour of his own professional advancement, to the pursuit of which the idiosyncrasies of such a wife as Laetitia would have constituted a formidable handicap. My unhappy aunt, serially spurned, threw herself by way of compensation into a career in letters, turning to good effect her early experience below stairs in the Morningside district of Edinburgh, and quickly establishing a reputation as the arbiter *nonpareil* of taste and good manners. Her weekly column in the *London Gazetteer* furnished the capital for a decade with its *vade-mecum* of fashionable mores. Her piece 'On gentlemanly conduct in the bed-chamber', for example, earned her the gratitude of many a Milady in aristocratic households.

I can now reveal that Laetitia was the anonymous benefactress whose secret munificence endowed the establishment of that august body, the Grand Medical Committee for Sorting Everything Out. From its very inception, the Grand Medical Committee attracted the participation of fashionable physicians and surgeons from every level and quarter of the profession, eager that their influence and power might extend not merely over the patients in their consulting rooms but as far as possible into the nation's social and political realms beside. So beguiling was the prospect that still to this day the Committee and its multitudinous sub-committees, working parties, steering groups and task forces exercise (I am told) an undiminished and almost hypnotic fascination for practitioners of the healing arts. With how wry a smile, therefore, must my aunt have discovered that prominent amongst the Grand Committee's founding luminaries were many who had turned their indifferent backs on her amorous blandishments. And how poignant, moreover, must have been her sense of frustration when copies of the Committee's early agendas, minutes and background papers were purloined from its secretariat and brought anonymously to her attention. For the issue

---

[3] Adapted from *Behind the lines*, Back Pages, *Brit. J. Gen. Pract.*, March 2003.

which, to the virtual exclusion of all others, dominated the discussions of the great and the good was the dress code to be observed during the Committee's meetings, a matter on which Laetitia (had she been consulted) could have provided sound and comprehensive guidance. I believe this was the irony that led her to compose, and then to place unpublished in a drawer, the essay which is hereinafter reproduced.

Miss Neighbour's health, it appears, was prematurely overwhelmed by a contagion contracted in the course of an ill-advised liaison south of the river, and the manuscript of her testamentary composition, 'On the wearing of hats', lay for three generations undiscovered in her escritoire. Fate, however, as I say, having now delivered it into my hands, I have made it an act of homage to prepare this her swansong for publication in these pages, hoping that the descendants in turn of her medical inamoratos may rue by proxy their forefathers' disdain which hastened her demise. If I correctly decipher her tear-smudged autograph, the text is preceded by the following dedication:

* * *

To those of the Medical Fraternity who would wear their Hats so low upon their Brow as to be blinded to the Hopes and Progress of Others; and to such the Author offers her best Counsel.

Choose one style of hat and remain faithful to it. It matters not whether your choice light upon fez or fedora, topper, trilby or tam-o'-shanter; the faithfulness is all. People will applaud you for it, and will, through your loyalty to one design, believe you to be a person of constancy and trustworthiness.

In size, colour and style your hat should complement your own capacities and bearing. An over-flamboyant or ill-matched hat may hint at vainglory and lay you open to surreptitious mockery.

Allow your hat, through regular wearing, to accommodate gently to the contours of your cranium. As the hat grows in your affection, so you likewise will grow in the affections of others. Replace it, when it grows shabby, only with another of identical design.

Choose a well-fitting hat. Nothing is more ridiculous than a hat so large as, by falling down over the brow, will obscure the wearer's countenance; nor one so small that the wearer, fearful it may blow off, is forever clutching it. A person corpulent in body or boisterous in nature may successfully sport a flamboyant, even an unfashionable, hat. Another, less generously endowed, courts foolishness unless a hat of more modest proportions is chosen.

It is commonly believed that, if too large a hat is habitually worn, the head of the wearer will expand to fill it. This is too uncertain a phenomenon to be relied upon, and when it occurs will startle and antagonise onlookers. Remember too that an over-large hat may cause difficulty in a strong wind. Do not jam it down all the harder on to your head, as it will catch the breeze like a sail, making progress perilous.

Yet, the regular wearing of a hat too small for a large head may engender an *hauteur* of the spirit, a compensatory conceit, attended by unwarranted hostility to others less lofty than yourself, on whose lesser brows it might have sat easy.

Wear only one hat at once. It may be that, out of doors or amongst strangers, a multiplicity of hats may pass almost unnoticed; but not so within doors or amongst familiars. To attempt the simultaneous wearing of more than one hat will cause pain in the neck, confusing some of the company, and enraging others.

It is ill-advised to take more than one hat into a meeting, and especially to change hats while it is in progress, however surreptitiously. The attempt to do so will assuredly be noticed and will call down ridicule upon you. Even should you possess a large collection of hats, you should resist the temptation to sport them in dizzy rotation. To onlookers, this suggests boastfulness or indecision.

Give thought, indeed, as to whether any hat need be worn at all. If attending a meeting where by common consent hats are *not* to be worn, leave your own outside, where it may nonetheless be admired on entering or leaving. Omitting to do so will provoke wearisome descriptions of hats your companions *could* have worn, to the detriment of the business of the day. In meetings where hats are customarily worn, should your hat be so large as to obscure the vision (or arouse the envy) of others, it is courteous to remove it.

When wearing a new hat for the first time, you should modestly draw attention to it, and graciously allow others to inspect and feel it, and appreciate its novelty, in order to gain confidence in its presence. It may happen that your new hat gives rise to much curiosity, even jealousy or resentment. In these circumstances you should on no account allow others to try it on, nor lend it. You should rather inform them where one of equal splendour is to be got for themselves; how you came by yours; and yet how exclusive it is, and how costly.

If on the other hand you possess no hat at all, you should not attempt a home-made one. The deception will be plain to see; and the sight of such a surrogate will inflame the passions of all those with bespoke millinery, or even ready-made.

A dilemma may arise if another person of the same company should come wearing a hat identical to your own. In this case, it is wisest for you and he to take up seats alongside each other; it is better to acknowledge the awkward-ness with a laugh than to sit on opposite aspects and affect ignorance of the duplication. Your companions will soon lose heart in their attempts to provoke division between you.

Take heed that to wear even your favourite hat on certain occasions – in bed, for example, or in an ale-house, or when travelling abroad – indicates instability, and may lead to that condition known to medical men as 'kapelophilia', a morbid addiction to the wearing of hats. Recovery from this affliction is prolonged and uncertain.

* * *

(And here my great-great-aunt's manuscript ends abruptly, for what reason I cannot tell. But is it coincidence that the casebook of Sir Jeremiah Q, physician, of Wimpole Street, records at about the time in question the paying of an unheralded house call to Downapeg Mansions and finding there a spinster needing urgent admission to the Bedlam Hospital for the Insane at St George's Fields, Southwark; and, in his further capacity as the Superintendent thereof, arranging the said admission most expeditiously?)

The Excalibur coefficient[4]

I'm a sucker for a half-decent aphorism. Aphorisms are the extra pepperoni on the deep-pan pizza of life. But statistics I'm *not* so fond of. Statistics are to the soul's free flight what muesli is to the back teeth.

A wise man once said – and I think it must have been a cousin of that other chap who made smart remarks about fishing – a wise man once said, 'Feed a man facts and you make him a clever fellow. Feed a man statistics and you make him a clever clogs.' I'd go further. The way I see it, to sign up for even the most basic '*Stats for toddlers*' course is to be set on a path that can lead eventually to a position of national power and influence.

I should know.

It's an ill-kept secret that I occasionally do a bit of moonlighting from my post here in the Department of Clinical Philosophy. For the past few years I have devoted a tithe of my leisure moments to the service of the RCGP, specifically as the Convenor of its Panel of MRCGP Examiners.[5] Well, the pension rights may not be much, but the company's fantastic.

The thing is, when I took on the post I rather under-estimated what was involved. I naïvely thought my duties would be roughly two in number. Firstly, I pictured myself drifting superfluously about the place, saying 'Carry on chaps' as the examination machinery purred smoothly away. I also knew it would be my job to answer the letters from unsuccessful candidates who wrote in claiming prejudice, incompetence or conspiracy on the part of their examiners as the sole reason for their failure. I swiftly developed a facility for replying in elegant variations on but a single theme, namely that the reason they failed the exam was that actually they didn't do well enough to pass. Strange but true.

It wasn't long before I found myself being invited *ex officio* to conferences of the great and the good on the world medical assessment scene. (Incidentally, for all their emphasis on outcome measures, the said great and good didn't seem above a bit of a nod in the direction of process, especially the digestive process. Isn't it odd that the most Spartan of academics nonetheless prefer to foregather where the sun and the Michelin stars shine most brightly – on the Isle of Capri, as it might be, but never the Isle of Dogs?)

Anyway, on one occasion there I was amongst all these exammy people, a guppy swimming with dolphins, hobnobbing with the David Newbles and the Sue Cases and the Dave Swansons and the Cees van der Vleutens[6] of this world. Then I noticed one poor outcast – an inoffensive-looking soul with sweet enough breath and a perfectly nice cardigan – to whom nobody ever spoke, whose glass at the drinks reception remained forever unreplenished, and whose upraised hand at question time never caught the chairman's eye. 'Who's that?' I asked one of the

---

[4] Adapted from *Education for General Practice* (2000), **11**, 467–71.
[5] Membership of the Royal College of General Practitioners – an examination taken by most doctors on or near completion of their three-year vocational training for general practice. It has four modules: a computer-marked multiple choice test of factual knowledge; a written paper testing applied knowledge and critical analysis; a video-based or simulated patient test of consulting skills; and an oral which tests decision-making and professional values.
[6] All acknowledged experts on the mathematics and statistics underpinning the assessment of doctors' clinical competence.

great (or it may have been the good). 'That,' came the pitying reply, 'is a man whose alpha is less than 0.8.' 'Ah,' I said.

We've got a new junior lecturer here in the Department of Clinical Philosophy, Greg by name, and when I got back he had the kettle on for coffee. 'What's alpha?' I asked him, pinching a surreptitious ginger nut.

Greg's face bore the look of a man who has found out the hard way that the toilet tissue lacks wet strength. 'You mean you don't know?' came the pitying reply. (In academic circles, I've noticed, a lot of replies seem to come pitying.)

'"Alpha" is a measure of internal consistency,' he told me. I was thinking the ginger nut's internal consistency was roughly that of concrete, but I suspected that wasn't what he meant. 'Go on,' I rashly invited him. And thus it came to pass that I received my first faltering lessons in validity and reliability and generalisability theory. I'd *heard* of generalisability, of course – who hasn't? But until then I'd just thought it sounded like that thing you do to amuse babies, where you flap your lips with a finger and make blobble-obble-obble noises.

'The alpha coefficient of a test,' Greg intoned as the afternoon dragged on, 'is the average of all possible split-half correlations.' 'Duh?' I said. 'Look,' he said. 'Think of it this way. Suppose you sit an exam with, say, 50 questions. You get given the result, your overall score on the test. You want to be sure that if you'd sat a similar test on another occasion you'd have got the same mark. We call that – ' (and he smirked a smirky smirk) ' – reliability.'

'But Greg,' I demurred, 'you can't get people to keep re-sitting an exam just to see if it's reliable. How do you get round that?'

'Easy,' he chortled. 'What you do is, you divide up your 50-question test and pretend it was two 25-question tests, and work out the correlation between the candidate's mark on the two halves. You could see what the candidate scored on questions 1 to 25, and see how it correlated with the mark on questions 26 to 50. If the test was perfect, the correlation would be 100%, same mark on each half. Or you could correlate scores on the odd-numbered questions and the evens. Or the scores on questions 2, 5, 8, 9, 14, 15, 18 ...'

'Yes thank you Greg,' I interjected, glancing at the clock.

I had indeed got the picture. Average out the correlations between an individual's scores on every possible half of a multi-item test, and you get a pretty good idea of whether the test is reliable. (Or at least internally consistent, which everybody agrees to pretend is the same thing.) Express that average as a figure between 0 and 1, and you've got the test's alpha coefficient. The great and the good, apparently, reckon that alpha has to be at least 0.8 before a test can hold its head up high and expect to get invited to a Palace garden party.

Signing the necessary requisition form, I sent Greg off to collect another packet of ginger nuts and slipped the old mind into free flow. Any exam, I now could see, tries to infer the whole from sampling a part. By quantifying a fraction of what candidates know, the examiner presumes to deduce the whole universe of their knowledge. The poet Blake, I reflected, wrote of seeing the world in a grain of sand. In that the world might be mapped point-to-point on to that tiny particle, and that therefore to know it completely is to know the entire universe, the grain of sand has an alpha coefficient of 1.

Thus it was that I developed some understanding of, even a fondness for, the statistical underpinning of that cruel sport known as setting an examination.

I learned not only about alphas but about kappas as well. In tests where not all candidates get asked the same questions, you can't have alphas. You have to have kappas, apparently. So, in the MRCGP, the video consulting skills module has a kappa (because each candidate submits their own choice of consultations to be assessed), whereas the written papers have alphas. To work out your kappa, you do actually put video tapes through the system twice, with different examiners, and see to what extent you get the same result on both times. Kappa (κ) can vary from +1 (complete agreement between both examiners) to −1 (total disagreement). A κ of 0 means random correlation, i.e. both examiners are guessing. Candidates and idealists get furiously agitated if ? is the tiniest bit less than +1. Examiners and realists, on the other hand, get ridiculously delighted if it's the tiniest bit better than 0. The great and the good, eternal pragmatists that they are, consider themselves lucky if κ is much above +0.4.

I learned about validity too. 'Validity' is statistician-speak for street cred. An exam has high 'content validity' if it tests the stuff that matters in the real world. It has 'construct validity' if the test methodology bears a passing resemblance to the way things are done in real life. So a 'single best answer' written question on the likely causes of green knee-caps has high construct validity, while a 'multiple true/false' test of communication skills does not. An assessment has 'face validity' if it looks plausible to the punters. It has 'predictive validity' if getting a good result on the test means you actually turn out OK in practice some years down track. (We don't yet have an entry test with good predictive validity which can be applied to medical school applicants, more's the pity. If we did, we could knock two years off vocational training.)

Checking the stats of the MRCGP, I in turn smirked a smirky smirk. Papers 1 and 2, its written and multiple choice components, regularly turn in alphas between 0.86 and 0.89, easily a match for any other assessment of primary care on the face of the earth. Alpha for the simulated surgery consulting skills module is 0.84. The video now delivers a kappa of +0.497. Brilliant! The great and the good raise their glasses in awestruck tribute.

But even as I learned about the value of statistical analysis in keeping an examination's feet on the ground, I found myself − cynic that I am − also noticing its down side. Somewhere, probably in Tibet, there may be a student of statistics whose devotion to the discipline is pure and incorruptible. But I haven't met him. In the hands of most of us mortals a half-decent statistic is not a torch-beam but a weapon. The advocates and adversaries of every method of assessment cudgel each other with numbers unmercifully. 'My alpha's bigger than *your* alpha,' some preening pundit will crow. 'Is that so?' replies a competitor, pityingly. 'Just wait till you see the size of my kappa!' An assessment's statistical indices are not simply tools to help it on its way towards fairness and reliability. Instead, they have become the instruments of intimidation, coercion, control, rivalry and bullying, with which protagonists in the assessment field seek to exalt their own endeavours and to belittle those of their academic opponents. An 'assessment civil war' threatens the United Kingdom's doctors, throwing professional satisfaction as we know it into the melting pot. And in that war, for all their protestations that analysis is merely the 'umble servant of truth, statisticians, albeit unwittingly, have become arms dealers.

It is we, by our disproportionate faith in psychometrics, who have corrupted them. It isn't the job of statisticians to agonise over the examiner-candidate relationship, or to run a help-line for the victims of numerical abuse. Mathematical probity is what statisticians peddle, and it's an honourable enough trade. We should not (as one of my favourite honest statisticians John Foulkes likes to remind me) mark down apples for not being pears. If we want to assess appliness but we've only got a set of pear-gauges, then we need something radically different.

But what?

Here in the Department we're working on this problem, and we think we may have the answer – ξ (xi), the Excalibur coefficient, so named after King Arthur's trusty sword.

The Excalibur coefficient, ξ, is a brand-new statistical index, an index of trustworthiness, i.e. a measure of the extent to which a candidate is 'safe in the examination's hands'. Think of it as a kind of kite-mark for assessment procedures.

We've provisionally identified five dimensions to the Excalibur coefficient, the first two of which we know about already. These are:

- validity
- reliability

and in addition:

- transparency
- equity
- jeopardy.

For an assessment to be trustworthy, we need satisfactory answers to the following questions, representing each dimension in turn.

- Does the test assess the right things and pass the right people ? (Validity, V)
- How sure can I, as a candidate, be that the result is right? (Reliability, R)
- Would I ever get to find out if it wasn't? (Transparency, T)
- If it wasn't, what would be the chances of getting something done about it? (Equity, E)
- What are the risks to me if the test failed me when I deserve to have passed? (Candidate Jeopardy, J_c)
- What are the risks to patients if the test passes me when I deserve to have failed? (Patient Jeopardy, J_p)

The formula for calculating the Excalibur coefficient, the index of trustworthiness, is:

$$\xi = \frac{VRTE}{(J_c + J_p)/2}$$

Each term in the formula needs its face washed and its hair brushed if it is to pass muster, and this is still very much 'work in progress'. Since they are all calculated differently according to the parameters of the particular assessment package being rated, all terms in the formula are scaled down and represented as a number between 0 and 1.

'Reliability' (R) is easy to quantify: this is where alpha and kappa come into their own. 'Validity' (V) isn't too hard in principle, either. It has two components – *content validity* (V_c), answering the question 'Does the test assess the right things?', and *predictive validity* (V_p), which tells you whether the right people pass. V_c could be the percentage of questions which, on being shown again to candidates after the exam, are greeted with comments such as, 'Fair enough, I ought to know that.' V_p could be the percentage of successful candidates who, five years later, have not been hauled up before the GMC for poor performance.

It's the soft fuzzy bits – Transparency, Equity and Jeopardy – that are hard to pin down with mathematics. Greg's been helping, of course. He's been down to the stationers no end of times collecting the flip-chart pads, Blu-tack, felt tips and highlighters with which the Department's creative space is festooned. I'm just a bit worried that he might think me ungrateful for his well-meant tuition in the rudiments of stats, implying, as this latest research does, that conventional wisdom isn't enough.

Our first attempts to put a figure on an exam's Transparency (T) involve estimating the percentage of all its marking and standard-setting procedures that are carried behind closed doors and out of the candidate's sight, transparency being the reciprocal of secrecy. Unfortunately, complete transparency ($T = 1$) would involve publishing the questions and marking schedules in advance, and getting candidates to mark their own answers. Now *there's* a radical thought ...

A measure of Equity (E) is given by the number and height of the various obstacles the exam authorities place in the way of a candidate who wants to challenge the result; in other words, how easy it is to trigger the appeals procedure. For $E = 1$, there would have to be an automatic and complete review of every failure. Now *there's* another radical thought ...

The Jeopardy (J) terms in the Excalibur coefficient address the 'Why bother and who cares?' dimension. J_c and J_p attempt to quantify the impact on candidate and patients respectively of a wrong result, i.e. of failing a candidate who deserved to pass, or passing a candidate who in the interests of patients or public should have failed. In truly high stakes tests, such as Summative Assessment or the GMC performance procedures, which determine whether a doctor is allowed to practise unsupervised, values of both Jeopardy components are high. The individual doodoo into which a wrongly-failed doctor is plunged is about as deep as the collective doodoo in which a wrongly-passing one can land the public. The Diploma in Verruca Studies on the other hand, which requires a 20 000-word dissertation and costs £1700 to sit, has a high J_c but a low J_p.

Wearing my MRCGP Convenor hat and using my trusty gut-weighted eyeball, I estimate values of the various terms for the MRCGP exam to be:

$$V = 0.8, R = 0.8, T = 0.4, E = 0.9, J_c = 0.5 \text{ and } J_p = 0.3$$

These give the exam an Excalibur coefficient of $2(0.8 \times 0.8 \times 0.4 \times 0.9)/(0.5 + 0.3)$, i.e.

$$\xi_{\text{MRCGP}} = 0.58$$

Could be better, of course, but not bad. You might like to try estimating ξ for some other assessment packages – medical final exams, for example, or the revalidation process for GPs. Anyway, if the MRCGP becomes a mandatory and therefore higher-stakes exam, values of J_c and J_p in the denominator would rise, lowering ξ. To maintain at least the present value of ξ, there would have to be compensatory increases in the exam's transparency and equity.

Now *there's* a radical thought . . .

9

When a new book is published . . .[1]

For over a decade, I reviewed books three or four times a year for what is known affectionately as 'the Green Journal', Radcliffe's publication of research, record and opinion in the world of primary care education. This chapter contains a few excerpts from these pieces. Some of the titles reviewed are by people whom I count as personal friends. This is not favouritism; I personally like the company of articulate mavericks, being one myself. And most authors are just that – articulate mavericks.

At the end of my last book review for the Green Journal, I wrote as follows:

> 'It's been my enormous pleasure since the inception of this Journal to indulge through these columns my love of books, respect for the travails of author-ship, and a search for a personal voice. I've tried to offset my ingrained distrust of authority with the wish to direct readers' attention to those quarters of the written landscape where inspiring visions and unexpected perspectives are to be glimpsed. The universal tragedy is that life, though lived forwards, is only understood backwards. Thinking and writing that aspire to buck this principle are always to be celebrated. Far too many published titles at the moment have no backbone. If general practice is under threat, it is not for the lack of "How to" information. What we need is a clearer and more intuitive grasp of "Why bother?" There is a danger that facts, advice and gold standards become, in the pursuit of them, the enemies respectively of truth, helpfulness and quality. It may be, as the millennium of scientism draws to a close, that these goals are more powerfully served obliquely and tangentially through the back door of fiction and drama than by the up-front hectoring of the literal-minded.'

Four books worth the effort?[2]

One of the nice things about a book reviewer's job is getting frequent parcels in the post from the medical publishing houses. The less pleasant thing, these last few months, has been opening them. *The Back-Of-A-Postage-Stamp Guide To This, Noddy's Colouring Book Of That, A Thousand And One Things You Never Wanted To*

---

[1] 'When a new book is published, read an old one.' Remark attributed to Samuel Rogers (1763–1855), English conversationalist, poet, and friend of greater poets, including Sheridan and Wordsworth.
[2] Adapted from *Postgraduate Education for General Practice* (1992), **3**, 84–7.

Know About The Other And Hoped No-one Would Ever Bother Telling You. Not a really good read amongst them. Just lists, facts, aide-mémoires and compendiums. No ideas. Nothing educational about education. Nothing by the general practice equivalent of Gandhi, or even Patience Strong. Not even anything new by Donald and Sally Irvine. Yet talk to our colleagues in medical education and you know there's no shortage of thoughtfulness or good ideas – just not in extended print.

If you talk to medical publishers about the market for general practice books, they tend to suck their teeth and put on a face like recession incarnate. GPs, it seems, never spend more than 35 old shillings on a book. Asked where books come from, they reply not 'from a bookshop', but 'off a drug rep'. And these same doctors (present company excluded, of course) who jib at 20 quid for hours of mental conversation with an author will quite happily fork out for a couple of CDs or a tournedos Rossini and all the trimmings. Why?

Various studies of trainees' learning strategies confirm that the reading habit is an endangered species. Wriggle as we may, the reason is not that books are too dear, too long, too numerous, too specialised or too often printed on paper. On the whole GPs don't buy many books because they don't read much. I find this terribly disappointing. I think – I *know* – that most of us have at one time or another found between the covers of a book a clarification, a stimulation, a falling-into-place, a falling-of-scales-from-the-eyes, and even the occasional inspiration. So why the present dearth of both medical restaurateurs and diners? To look at the current publishers' lists you'd think that all GPs can stomach is the literary equivalent of the pot noodle, while all that trainees will touch is a pap of nutritionally-complete minced factlets, pre-digested to enhance their performance in the MRCGP exam. Part of it must still be the beleaguered feelings engendered by the paroxysms within the NHS, which have sapped people's desire to absorb any more ideas and information than they absolutely have to[3].

To emphasise the difference between what's all too common and all too rare, let's look at two examples of books intended to be used as a summary or compendium of general practice – its clinical, organisational and conceptual aspects, doctors in their consulting rooms for the use of. *Aids to General Practice*[4] is the latest, in the words of its author, to summarise 'the essentials of general practice'. Written in the form of lists and tables, much of it 'should be committed to memory by any candidate approaching the MRCGP examination'. Asthma, it would seem, is under-diagnosed. The duties of the reception staff include manning the reception desk. Health visitors have a broad job description, while the practice nurse is a key member of the primary healthcare team. Strewth! The author has done a perfectly respectable and comprehensive job within the format imposed, presumably, by his editors. What bothers me is that anyone should want him to.

The two pocket-sized *Oxford Handbooks, of Clinical Medicine*[5] and *of Clinical Specialties*[6], are, on the other hand, brilliant. I keep them by my chair and refer to

---

[3] Editing in 2004 (under a Labour administration) this text written in 1992 (under its Tory predecessor), I sadly didn't feel any need to explain this bit. Plus ça change.
[4] Mead M (1990) *Aids to general practice (2nd edition)*. Churchill Livingstone, Edinburgh.
[5] Hope RA, Longmore JM, Moss PAH and Warrens AN (1989) *Oxford handbook of clinical medicine (2nd edition)*. Oxford University Press, Oxford.
[6] Collier JAB, Longmore JM and Harvey JH (1991) *Oxford handbook of clinical specialties (3rd edition)*. Oxford University Press, Oxford.

them at least three times a day in full and unashamed view of patients. The level of clinical information is pitched exactly right, up to date and exhaustive, while the style is a masterly balance between textbook compression and fireside philosophy. A trainee reading the general practice section will effortlessly and painlessly absorb the equivalent of 73 hours of tutorials. I quote (and feel genuinely moved as I do so):

> 'When Miss Phelps' baby dies she is not a medical problem; she is not an obstetric problem; she is not even a psychiatric problem – she is Miss Phelps. And the doctor who specialises in Miss Phelps is (or ought to be) her GP ... The newcomer to general practice might conclude that GPs spend most of their time setting up primary care teams, conducting audits, loading programs of prevention onto their computers, engaging in performance review, delegating to the team, and, in those few cases where actually consulting personally then following this with a long period of video-taped consultation analysis. Until very recently general practice has not felt the need for any of the above. What has brought these activities to the forefront is that we are awakening to a world where there are limits to the success of technological medicine ... This is the great challenge of general practice – to foster in oneself an equal love of, and an excellence in, both the technological and the personal realm.'

I wish I'd written that. There's something rare and precious in it – gold as against brass, Mahler against Mantovani. Every consulting room, and every doctor at every career stage, should have the *Handbook* set, and I don't say that lightly.

Another area where we are (all right, where I am) always looking for fresh insights is the Balint-dominated territory of the doctor-patient relationship. For my money, the most uplifting contribution to the recent literature in this field rejoices in the off-putting title of *Mutative Metaphors in Psychotherapy – The Aeolian Mode*[7]. It's no longer new, but it's fresh and (that word again) inspirational, giving a sense that a crucial horizon is not so far away as we thought it was. It's about stories, about metaphors and images, about how the therapeutic ear can accustom itself to hear a universal narrative within the individual tale of the individual's tragedy. If the following quotations hold out to you any prospect of insight, you will love this book:

> 'The image has touched the depths before it stirs the surface.'
> 'Therapy is concerned with a story so disturbing that, however painful the telling, it must be attempted.'
> 'Frontiers of consciousness beyond which words fail, though meanings still exist.'
> 'What is concealed in what is proclaimed.'
> 'There are colours other than black and white – and I think I ought to see them.'

If you half believe that medicine's about everything except what's in the textbooks, treat yourself, astound yourself – get into the Aeolian Mode. You've probably been in it already without realising.

---

[7] Cox M and Theilgaard A (1987) *Mutative metaphors in psychotherapy – the Aeolian mode.* Tavistock Publications, London.

The Doctor's Communication Handbook[8]

You get the impression that, to some authors, writing about general practice feels much the same as truffle-hunting must do to the pig. Not an ordinary pig, you understand, such as is happy in muck. A pig with attitude. A pig with aspirations. A pig in the wrinkle of whose brow hauteur hopes to pass for breeding. A pig who, although reduced to grubbing for a living, goes home at night to a sty crammed with alabaster busts of the late Sir Porker and the thirteenth Baron Saddleback. A pig, in short, who can just about cope with dirtying its feet with the mud of authorship as long as it can dab a spot of Chanel behind its ears to waft a faint protest to the workaday world, 'Oh that it should come to this!' Disdainful.

And again: you get the impression that, to some casual observers, general practice must appear virtually indistinguishable from golf. The skilled practitioner of both activities knows this to be no sneer, but actually a rather sharp insight. The essence of each is the same rather compulsive stalking of something that is wilful, immune to threat and entreaty, but desperately and disproportionately important; the same frustration of no sooner lighting on one option – one club, one line to the hole – than having seven others suggest themselves; the same ungainly contortions of mortal flesh attempting to approximate itself to the elegant ideals of the demigods; and above all, the same recurring crushing awareness that the technical difficulties are as moonlight unto sunlight compared with the internal invisible demonic battle against doubt and self-criticism. Anguished.

And so to my good friend, the golf-renouncing truffle-eschewing Peter Tate, formerly one third of the *et al.* in the Pendleton classic[9] and now sole author of *The doctor's communication handbook*, I send a copy of Dorothy Parker's telegram to an actress friend, newly delivered after an ill-concealed pregnancy: 'Good work. We all knew you had it in you.'

Bravo Pete. The fruit of your loins manages to be both beautiful and the spitting image of its dad. I've always thought single author books had more oomph, and this one is an uninhibited paean of good communication by someone who reckons talking with patients to be an art form and not an academic discipline. I'm sure it *wasn't* written this way, but you'd think Peter had taken his favourite medical student, his favourite trainee and his favourite godchild, and entertained them over dinner and long into the night with the Dictaphone switched on. As a result, his book has a fluency and an immediacy which more than compensates for the occasional gung-ho moment, e.g. 'The GP's primary duty is to protect patients from hospital medicine'.

There are some lovely cameos breathing life into – yes, you guessed it – Ideas, Concerns and Expectations[10], health beliefs, and a few new friends such as the

---

[8] Tate P (1994) *The doctor's communication handbook*. Radcliffe Medical Press, Oxford. Adapted from *Education for General Practice* (1994), **5**, 103–6. This review was of the first edition; the fourth edition (2002) is now available.

[9] Pendleton D, Schofield T, Tate P and Havelock P (1984) *The consultation: an approach to learning and teaching*. Oxford University Press, Oxford. (Known to the vocational training world as 'Pendleton *et al.*'.)

[10] The triad of Ideas, Concerns and Expectations (ICE) encapsulates what the patient brings to the consultation and hopes to get out of it. ICE has become so much quoted as a mnemonic as to become the clichéd slogan of every doctor who wishes to appear patient-centred.

'locus of control'. The classic Pendletonian analysis is still here, with its seven tasks recast into a subdivided five. Pete's chapter on consultation strategies and skills is full of good ideas, some of them his own:

> 'Closing the notes can signal the end of the consultation. Wearing a dinner jacket tends to speed things up a bit, but cannot be used too often. Taking the chair away is a last resort.'

Quite a few sacred cows lie bleeding after Tate has motored by. Here he is on 'the current craze for giving life-style advice':

> 'To come to your doctor with a cold and be told to stop smoking, lose weight, have your cervix smeared, your breasts examined and your cholesterol measured, and, to boot, that you can't have any cough mixture prescribed for you, may to a large section of the community be profoundly unsatisfying. However, the profession as a whole, by a majority verdict, would probably consider this good practice.'

And on people who believe themselves to be in charge of their own health destiny and who:

> '... will not have an aluminium pot in the house for fear of Alzheimer's and who are to be found sweating in health food shops rummaging for the elixir of life having just jogged five miles to get there. (These people) tend to get very cross if they get ill. To spend 20 years abstaining from the good things in life to keep one's cholesterol below 5, and then still have a coronary at 55, makes for a very unhappy and disillusioned human being.'

Or on the totally patient-centred doctor:

> '... probably another dangerous creature. Patients ... don't expect a laid-back hippie to let them do all the talking, planning and managing for themselves.'

That's the Pete Tate I know and love, the iconoclastic epicure with the external locus of control who reckons that 'in this life God gives you a certain number of heartbeats and I'm buggered if I'm wasting any of mine running round in bloody circles on wet Sunday mornings!'[11]

The abiding impression is of a wise and compassionate doctor with affection bordering on love for the work he does and the people he cares for, and who longs to have his pupils appreciate the same warmth and closeness. The book is engaging, and does indeed engage; and an engaged reader is more than half wedded to the author's passion. Again, bravo.

---

[11] Personal communication, *circa* 1993. I should, in the interests of scrupulous honesty, report that, in 2001, Tate underwent an almost religious conversion to the Atkins diet, which by a series of misfortunes – described in *Education for Primary Care* (2003), **14**, 251–3 – almost cost him his remaining heartbeats. This should not, however, be taken to undermine the validity of his views on what many MRCGP exam candidates, in an unsuspectingly accurate malapropism, refer to as 'health prevention'.

The Death of Humane Medicine[12]

First, a song.

> 'The flowers that bloom in the spring, Tra-la,
> Breathe promise of merry sunshine.'

Thus, in Gilbert and Sullivan's *Mikado*, chortled Nanki-Poo as, with the betrothal of the ghastly Katisha to the luckless Ko-Ko, his own prospects of a life in thrall to ugliness receded.

It feels as if in my book reviews over the last year or two I've alternated between lamentation and envy. Lamentation that much of the output of UK medical publishers has of necessity consisted of first aid manuals offering advice on how to survive the intellectual famine and second-hand car dealer values of the new NHS. And envy that authors from other systems of primary care, notably in the USA, still preserve sufficient uncontaminated zeal to write about the things that really matter, like people and relationships and feelings, about good practice and bad, right and wrong. For thoughtfulness doesn't easily survive in a moral Ice Age[13], and creativity has been easily trampled under the feet of marauding bureau-brats.

But suddenly the Spring book lists are full of promise! There's a faint whiff of something heady in the air. Could it be nostalgia? Or adolescence? No matter; when it comes to contemplating yet more changes to the NHS, wistfulness and rebelliousness are often one and the same thing.

First up is an invigorating publication from a house new to me – the Social Affairs Unit. The SAU is a charitable research and educational trust 'committed to the promotion of lively and wide-ranging debate on social affairs'. And some. The particular title that caught my eye was Petr Skrabanek's last book *The death of humane medicine*, subtitled, as if that wasn't polemical enough, *and the rise of coercive healthism*[14].

I never got to meet Petr Skrabanek before his untimely death in 1994. I regret this, for much the same reasons that it would have been nice to have seen a safely-caged sabre-toothed tiger in the flesh. If you've read his *Follies and fallacies in medicine*[15] you'll know that Skrabanek is the intellectual successor to Ivan ('The medical establishment has become a major threat to health') Illich[16]. In *The death of*

---

[12] Adapted from *Education for General Practice* (1995), **6**, 181-5.
[13] This was written in 1995. My impression is that, in the last few years, books on general practice published in the UK have moved away from the formulaic and have recaptured some energy and originality, whereas transatlantic primary care titles have deteriorated in the opposite direction. Whether this correlates with the advent of a new moral Ice Age in the USA is for the reader to say; I couldn't possibly comment.
[14] Skrabanek P (1994) *The death of humane medicine and the rise of coercive healthism*. The Social Affairs Unit, London.
[15] Skrabanek P and McCormick J (1989) *Follies and fallacies in medicine*. Tarragon Press, Glasgow. Typical is this definition: 'Scepticaemia: an uncommon generalised disorder of low infectivity. Medical school education is likely to confer life-long immunity.'
[16] Ivan Illich (1926–2002). Vienna-born Catholic priest, polymath, ascetic and intellectual. In a series of books between 1971 and 1982 he conducted a sustained, but far from vinegary, campaign against the institutions of the industrialised world. He particularly targeted the professions, including medicine and teaching, for undermining individual resourcefulness by cultivating dependency and a monopoly of supply. The line quoted opens and summarises his 1975 book *Medical nemesis*. Calder & Boyars, London.

humane medicine he confronts and (to my satisfaction at least) demolishes 'the dangerous ideology of "the health of the nation" '.

Which of us – when perfectly healthy people turn up in a panic because their BUPA health screen has revealed a blood pressure of 122/81, or when the first conversation with a new patient degenerates into sanctimonious twaddle about exercise and All-Bran – has not felt a frisson of resentment? Who – seeing the fervour with which some (often young) colleagues bang on about cholesterol and insult the obese – has not wished we had at our fingertips the facts to jolt them out of their self-deluding credulity? And who – after pocketing the money for hitting, by hook or by crook, the latest Department of Health targets – has not sidled over to the hand-basin to wash away the tacky taint of the pork barrel?

For we have watched with mounting dismay as the epidemiologists and advisory committees and health promotionists have built themselves an Imperial palace of grandiose proportions, and set it in formal gardens of beguiling precision. But the Emperor has no clothes; the palace is made of ginger-bread and built upon sand; and the immaculate grounds are just crying out to have a coach and horses driven through their midst. Petr Skrabanek can not only supply such a coach and horses; he can drive them with verve and accuracy, and be off and away and laughing before the defenders have cleared the sleep from their eyes.

Skrabanek structures his diatribe in three sections. The first he summarises thus:

> 'The pursuit of health is a symptom of unhealth. When this pursuit is no longer a personal yearning but part of state ideology, it becomes a symptom of political sickness; ... The medical profession, particularly its public health branch, provides the required theoretical underpinning of healthism – the doctrine of life-stylism, according to which most diseases are caused by unhealthy behaviour ... There is a point beyond which a liberal profession turns into a disabling profession, beyond which the balance between personal autonomy and medical paternalism is lost and society starts sliding towards a nanny state, and then further into techno-facism ... Medicine has no mandate to be meddlesome.'

In his second section, *Lifestylism*, Skrabanek calls the roll of today's sacred cows – dietary obsession, joyless exercise, cardiovascular 'risk factors', screening, regular check-ups – and one by one despatches them. Whenever the usual suspects are rounded up – promiscuity, fatty foods, alcohol and secondary smoking – he provides them with alibis galore. It would be scurrilous, were not his knowledge of the published (and sometimes the suppressed) research literature so impeccable.

Finally Skrabanek alerts us to the way medicine, albeit often unwittingly, has been coerced to carry out the will of politicos whose motives are anything but altruistic.

> 'The ways of implementing healthist politics include the substitution of health education by health-promotion propaganda; ... the coercion of general practitioners, through financial inducements, to act as agents of the state; the presentation of the politically corrupt science of healthism as objective knowledge ... Healthist authorities are not directly accountable to the public. They operate in a moral vacuum. Their power is, in practice, uncontested because of the legitimacy they have spuriously borrowed from medicine and science and their concerned beneficence. Their potential for harm is unassessed.'

Alleluia! It's Spring.

An irascible fairy[17]

Oh, isn't it infuriating when it's on the tip of your tongue? You know who I mean, the irascible fairy in *Peter Pan*. I'm probably misremembering the plot, but the one who got a bit tetchy with the Darling children when they were making such heavy weather of learning to fly, when all they had to do was to think lovely wonderful thoughts, wriggle their shoulders and let go. What *was* her name? Tinkerbell, that's it. That's who Iona Heath reminds me of. Tinkerbell.

Iona's John Fry Trust Fellowship lecture on *The mystery of general practice* has been published as a monograph[18], and I think it's terrific.

The eponymous 'mystery' is not why anybody should want to do general practice, but rather the inarticulate nature of the fundamental transaction between doctor and patient. Iona Heath is one of nature's useful irritants, one of the oyster-bed's pearl-inducing grains of sand. Her book is unashamed rhetoric, but rhetoric very much to the point; that point being to work up a head of resistance to some of the nonsenses and outrages being perpetrated on general practice in the name of logic.

Iona takes as her starting point value conflicts such as those between the doctor's role as advocate for the individual and that of social guardian of distributive justice, ensuring fair access by all too limited resources. But there is no danger here of passionate matters being presented dispassionately. Poets, novelists, philosophers – all are her desk-fellows. She enlists the poet Shelley to describe the injustice whereby 'The rich grind the poor into abjectness and then complain that they are abject'. She is inspired by Arthur Kleinman's observation that 'The physician's training encourages the dangerous fallacy of over-literal interpretation of accounts best understood metaphorically'. 'We must make available the benefits of scientific medicine,' she writes, 'but mitigate its dangers through an understanding of anthropology, biography, poetry, myth, philosophy and politics.' Anthropology and biography assist empathy; poetry and myth suggest the language to communicate our understanding; and philosophy and politics prompt us to be effective partisans on behalf of our patients.

A key role for the GP, Iona reminds us, is 'to serve as a witness to the patient's experience of illness and disease'. Since reading this, I've found it genuinely helpful. Within the last week, when the occasional patient has poured forth a torrent of insolubilities, I've been able to tell myself that what is wanted from me is not another game of 'Yes, but …' It's enough for me just to hear, for it to be known that I have heard, to aspire to be nothing more than a witness. And I've become very calm.

We doctors are relatively late entrants and reluctant recruits into the ranks of those who search for meaning in life's vicissitudes. Bards and priests, story-tellers and mystics have all been there ahead of us; and if we try to elbow them aside with cries of 'Let me through, I'm a doctor' we shouldn't be surprised if sometimes we get our comeuppance.

---

[17] Adapted from *Education for General Practice* (1996), **7**, 89–93.
[18] Heath I (1995) *The mystery of general practice*. The Nuffield Provincial Hospitals Trust, London.

10

Two sacred cows

All civilisations have their sacred cows – beliefs or principles whose truth is taken for granted, questioned only by heretics or the feeble-minded. General practice has a few sacred cows of its own: the primary healthcare team, for example; the sanctity of the doctor-patient relationship; independent contractor status.

It seems to me that one hallmark of a thriving civilisation is to know a sacred cow when we see one. This is not necessarily to kill it or desanctify it, but simply to recognise it for what it is – a working assumption, a convenient and pragmatic way of doing things, not a revelation of divine truth. Sacred cows are not to be blindly worshipped, but rather milked of their nourishment and, if barren, put out to grass.

This section faces down two such sacred cows in the field of contemporary medical thought. The first – evidence-based medicine – has been greeted with much garlanding and strewing of petals in its path. And why not? Who could gainsay such a common sense message as 'base what you do for patients on the best available evidence'? Well, there are some – and this book contains plenty of references to them who – maintain that much of what is important in personalised care is invisible to the double blind trial. Where, we might ask, is the evidence that evidence-based care is better than any other sort? After all, it has long been recognised that if you make a determined effort to screen and treat everybody for borderline hypertension, whatever vascular disease you prevent in the community overall has to be offset, for many unpredictable individual patients, against anxiety, hypochondriasis and cardiac neurosis.

The second piece is a protest at the current supremacy of a particularly insidious way of introducing control into professional practice – circular thinking, as exemplified by the audit cycle. There are some fallacies in circular thinking. It can lead ultimately to a steady state which may actually deter the creative evolutionary processes that civilisation depends on for its advance.

On the basis of the evidence[1]

One of the few drawbacks to my appointment to the Radcliffe Armchair of Clinical Philosophy is that my busy programme of contemplative research sometimes causes me to fall a little behind in my reading of the current literature. But unanswered questions and unquestioned assumptions abound on all sides, and – if evidence-based medicine is ever to be more than a slogan – they must each be recast as a research opportunity and the truth winkled out. Take a recent case in point.

[1] Adapted from *Education for General Practice* (2000), **11**, 228–32.

Lately, I've been watching the decorators give a lick of magnolia to the department's side corridor, where Greg, one of my junior lecturers, has his cubbyhole. Determined to turn even so banal an event as this to advantage, I conducted a little study whose conclusions (to anticipate a paper in preparation for the *J. Soc. Blind. Obv.*) can be summarised as follows:

1   Paint dries at a rate inversely proportional to the fascination of the observer.
2   The fascination of the observer is directly proportional to the number of passers-by likely to brush up against it while it's still wet.

From this it follows that, if you want your paint to dry quickly, you should keep the public well away. Conversely, if a casual bystander happens to get his kicks from seeing a perfectly good jacket ruined, the paint will never dry. The research evidence is quite conclusive, and the sooner the Royal College of Painters and Decorators updates its protocols in the light of it the smarter the nation's corridors will be.

Anyway, given that my time has been occupied with these weighty matters, you'll perhaps forgive the fact that my slush pile of unread books, journals and reprints had reached a height of eight foot six. So no sooner had the painters moved on than I settled down and made a start on *The Observer* of Sunday, January 5th 1800. Yes, I know − 1800, and I'm sorry, but it was very slow-drying paint, OK? My eye was caught by a notice[2], towards the bottom of column three on the front page, published by Dr John Mather, Member of the Royal College of Physicians, London. In it the said Doctor Mather *'respectfully informs his Friends and the Public, that he now resides at No. 25, King Street, Soho.'* Doubtless it was a respectable address two centuries ago. Moreover, the good doctor continues, *'He cannot but think it his duty to adopt any Remedy which attentive Observation and Experience assure him is eminently calculated to relieve the afflicted, in a variety of Diseases, especially those of a tropical kind.'*

So far, so evidence-based. But blow me if his small ad didn't continue, *'He therefore purposes to add to the usual Remedies, Dr PERKINS's METALLIC TRACTORS, which probably may most successfully be applied by a Medical hand. Though they do no harm even where they do no good, he has sufficient reason to believe that they possess great powers, when a proper discrimination is made as to the nature of the case.'*

My finely-tuned researcher's mind swiftly formulated several questions. What in the name of goodness are Dr Perkins' metallic tractors? Why might only a medical hand best apply them? And, most intriguingly, what 'Observation and Experience', what 'sufficient reason' and 'proper discrimination' had led Dr Mather to invest several farthings in publicly endorsing them?

I touched the bell-push and summoned Greg. 'If you've nothing better to do, Greg,' I suggested, 'see if there's anything about this Perkins chappie and his tractors in the data base.'

He was back, jubilant, within the hour. 'Nothing on Medline, Boss,' he reported, 'but I found something in the dictionary. See here: Perkins' metallic tractors − "a device invented by Elisha Perkins, an American physician who died in 1799, consisting of a pair of pointed rods of different metals, e.g. brass and steel, which

[2] *The Observer*, No. 420 (5th Jan. 1800). Publ. Joseph Watson, No. 169 The Strand, Two Doors Westward of Surry-Street, London. (No, honestly!)

were believed to relieve rheumatic or other pain by being drawn or rubbed over the skin. The usage is now Obs. except Hist."[3] What does that mean, "Obs. except Hist."? Obstetric except histological?'

Oh dear. You just can't get the staff.

Luckily at that moment I fell into the state which contemplative researchers know as creative delirium, but which to the untutored eye looks like sleep, and which is usually rendered in film by a ripple dissolve to denote a dream-like flashback to a bygone time ...

... in which I see Penelope, Lady Gullible, reclining in night apparel (though the bright daylight of the 19th century's first Sunday morning streams through the windows of her Piccadilly bedchamber) upon a chaise longue, and sipping a bitter medicinal decoction of willow bark. She hears footsteps approaching across the landing, and the door is rapped with the knuckles of a servile hand. 'Breakfast, my lady,' says a lackey, entering with a tray. 'I have brought you the newspaper, and a French letter.'

Her ladyship's superior education reminds her that it is far too early in the century for this line to be funny, so she merely opens the envelope, recognising with a quickening pulse the hand of her old admirer, the late Marquis de Condorcet.

'*Having been dead these last six years,*' she reads, '*I just thought I'd write. Here in France the Enlightenment proceeds apace. The weather is fine, and the improvement of medical practice, which will become more efficacious with the progress of reason, will mean the end of infectious and hereditary diseases and illnesses brought on by climate, food, or working conditions. It is reasonable to hope that all other diseases may likewise disappear as their distant causes are discovered[4]. How are the rheumaticks, by the way? Hoping this finds you as it leaves me, yours philosophically, Marie-Jean-Antoine-Nicolas.*'

Lady Gullible turns next to her newspaper and reads, wide-eyed, Dr Mather's announcement. She is much taken with his careful emphasis on Observation and Experience. She dares to hope that the unrequited ache in the very marrow of her bones, the nameless longings that wrack her frame, might yet yield to the powers of Dr Perkins's metallic tractors. What would the Marquis advise?, she asks herself, and sends her servant to command Dr Mather's attendance that very day.

Dr Mather is of a certain age, reassuring, kind, with a bedside demeanour that encourages the imparting of confidences. 'Do you think the tractors may relieve me?' Lady Penelope asks him.

'Do not doubt it,' he replies, and the look of earnest concern on his face convinces her.

'Good Doctor Mather,' cries Lady Penelope, 'you are your own guarantee; I am persuaded.'

'If then your Ladyship would unfasten her robe, to allow the Perkinsian device access to the troublesome parts ...' The metal probes are cold as they caress her skin, but soon she feels an encouraging warmth suffusing her aching limbs and gladdening her soul. 'Do you feel the benefit?' the doctor enquires.

'I do, I do,' she breathes. And indeed she does; for when a commotion on the stairs heralds the arrival, breathless, of her husband Sir Percival in high choler, it is with unusual serenity that she greets him.

---

[3] *The Oxford English Dictionary (2nd edition)* (1989) 'Thro' to 'Unelucidated', p. 346. Oxford University Press, Oxford.
[4] Quoted in Porter R (1997) *The greatest benefit to mankind.* Harper Collins, London.

'Devil take your good mornings, madam,' snarls the knight. And, turning to the flustered Dr Mather, he charges him, 'Explain, Sir, if you can, upon what pretext you make so free with my wife's person!'

'Well,' Dr Mather begins, 'these tractoration rods are the height of medical fashion, being imported from the Americas, where they have gained approval in the best houses of Baltimore and Boston for the relief of divers langours and stiffnesses ...'

'Be that as it will,' interrupts Sir Percival, intrigued despite himself, 'but by what means?'

'By the electrical power of the twin metals, combining the stiffness of steel with the softness of copper, each drawing forth its reciprocal quality from the afflicted muscles and galvanising ...'

'And your evidence for their efficacy?'

Dr Mather is on firmer ground. 'I have here signed testimonials from Lady Fleeceworthy, Lady Heartsink, the Honourable Mrs Simpleton, the Countess of Dupe, the Duchess of Pushover ...'

At the last name Sir Percival harrumphs, for he knows the Duchess better under the name of 'Sweetlings'. 'Doubtless your patient is advised a further dose of the Perkinsian remedy,' he says. Dr Mather nods. 'Then,' says Sir Percival triumphantly, 'let it be your assistant and not yourself who applies it, so that we may see whether the tractors retain their effectiveness in other, less familiar, hands.'

Thus, a week later, it is young Doctor Scoffie who, unsmiling and peremptory, attends Lady Gullible as *locum tenens* for the charismatic Dr Mather. The previous day Scoffie has lunched with Erasmus Darwin, a more fashionable physician, who has offered him a guinea a year more than Mather is paying. Darwin has turned Scoffie's head with the notion that lower forms of life inherently and through their own energy transmute into higher ones, and the young man is minded to put this possibility to the test in the laboratory of his own career. Already he has begun to think of his erstwhile mentor, his teachings, his beliefs, his techniques and his patients as obstacles to his own advancement. And so today it is abstractedly and to little avail that Dr Scoffie prods and jabs Lady Penelope's cringing limbs with Elisha Perkins' invention. Her Ladyship finds Dr Scoffie's lack of conviction infectious, and, betrayed, she unceremoniously sends him and his metallic tractors packing.

And then I must have stirred fitfully in my creative delirium, for, with one of those breathtaking *non sequiturs* one finds in dreams and radio phone-ins, I found myself playing a scene in which the great detective assembles all the suspects in the library and reveals The Truth.

'Before we pass the judgement of history on Dr Perkins' metallic tractors,' I hear myself saying, 'let us review the evidence for and against them. Or rather,' I continue, looking hard at each witness in turn, 'let us review what it is that each of you will allow to be considered as evidence.

'Dr Mather, you are an honest man. To you, the plain word of a colleague whom you regard as trustworthy, the illustrious Dr Perkins, is sufficient evidence. The letters of testimonial from some of your patients, though flattering, do not increase your enthusiasm for tractoration, any more than the withholding of any such endorsement by others who have found no benefit would diminish it. A natural philosopher such as the Marquis of Condorcet would have looked upon you as a true scion of the Enlightenment, believing as you do that the struggle for improvement in the human condition need not wait upon explanatory detail. "Let us have vision, and theory, and expectation first," he would say, "and let the facts follow when they may."

'My Lady, you by contrast would happily rely on the evidence of your own experience, were it not so contradictory. The benefit you derived from the tractors in Dr Mather's hands was just as real as their failure in those of Dr Scoffie. I believe that, had your husband's suspicions not intervened, you would have been cured – though not, perhaps, through the agency of Elisha Perkins' invention. You had done better to persist with the decoction of willow bark.

'Sir Percival, you are a suspicious, duplicitous and ungenerous bully. No, do not raise your fist to me, Sir, for these qualities are in fact meritorious aspects of your nature, which will flush out the true worth of the tractors, whereas the credulity of others will allow it concealment. Sorrowfully, however, your hasty dismissal of your wife's preferred physician has denied her a cure, cost Dr Mather his reputation, and made a turncoat of his pupil. I hope only that your satisfaction has not exacted too high a price.

'As for you, young Scoffie, well may you hang your head in shame. The truth, to you, is a flighty thing – Mather may have it today, Darwin tomorrow. It is a Proteus, taking now this form, now that, according to the prevailing wind. And see how your indifference has confused Lady Gullible. While you were Dr Mather's apprentice, did you not owe him some loyalty, some obligation to apply his beloved tractors with at least some semblance of conviction, if only for his patient's sake?'

Scoffie looks so wretched that I hasten to comfort him. 'Yet of all those here assembled, you have come closest in understanding. Evidence does not always build into facts. Facts are not always certainties, and certainty is not always the best foundation for usefulness.'

As I warmed to my theme the characters seemed to fade, leaving me, as it were, preaching to an empty room. 'How do we decide which kind of truth is the right one for the moment?' I soliloquised. 'We take in experiences and convert them into different versions of truth, much as we ingest food and turn it into tissues and organs. The scientific kind of truth has no monopoly, and must compete for survival with all the other kinds – pragmatic, artistic, symbolic, emotional and metaphorical truth – in an evolutionary struggle that Erasmus Darwin's grandson Charles will shortly describe. Truth is whatever works, whatever enables the influence and value systems of its possessor to survive and to prevail . . .'

The next thing I knew, Greg was standing over me, fanning me back into consciousness with a copy of the *BMJ*. 'I think I've just had a bad dream,' I told him. 'Evidence-based medicine as we know it was in the melting-pot. You can put that journal back in the library. Under "Fiction".'

He departed, leaving the *Oxford English Dictionary* still open at 'Perkins' metallic tractors'. I couldn't resist a glance. Regular readers of the *OED* will know that each definition is followed by a chronological series of quotations, charting the evolution of the entry's usage. They made, in this case, an interesting summary of the rise and fall of this quaint episode in the history of quackery. I quote:

> 1798 C C Langworth: 'A view of the Perkinean electricity', or, 'An inquiry into the influence of metallic tractors.'

1801 E Darwin:	'With the supposed existence of ghosts or apparitions, witchcraft, vampyrism and American tractors, such theories must vanish.'
1803 Fessende:	'Terrible tractoration; a poetical petition against galvinizing trumpery and the Perkinistic institution.'
1825 Southey:	'His prayers may cure just as well as tractors or animal magnetism.'
1880 Library of Universal Knowledge (New York):	'A Perkinsian institution was established in London for the benefit of the poor.'
1885 Whittie:	'Perkins, in drawing out diseases with his metallic tractors, was quite as successful as modern "faith and mind" doctors.'

I wonder what examples a future edition will choose to illustrate its entries on 'lipid-lowering agents'. Or 'adult learning', say, or 'the doctor-patient relationship'.

On disinventing the wheel[5]

To those of you who were kind enough to send me good wishes following my recent trauma may I say thank you, and yes, I'm pretty much recovered. Greg himself, the rising star of my Department of Clinical Philosophy, is of course mortified to have been the instrument of my injury. The headaches are less frequent and the tyre marks on my rump have all but faded, but I do still get flashbacks.

Almost the last thing I remember is coming in early one morning with good intentions and a pot of white paint, having it in mind, as a gesture friendship, to paint Greg's name on his slot in the departmental bike rack. Leadership, in my philosophy, should be 'bottom up'; and on this occasion, as I bent to my task, fate took me literally. Viewed upside down from between my knees, something resembling the Angel of the North hurtled towards me and, in the split second before impact, resolved itself into Greg astride his boneshaker, hands clutched to his mouth and legs akimbo.

I've already had occasion in these pages to refer to the insight-favouring properties of semi-consciousness. The chemist Kekule, you will recall, sussed the structure of the benzene ring when, nodding post-prandially in his fireside chair, he fancied in the flickering flames a snake, which took its own tail into its mouth. With me this time it was wheels. The concussing darkness which overwhelmed me seemed filled to superfluity with wheels, spinning and skidding and generally getting where they had no business to be.

The philosopher's calling is to distil profundity from the humdrum, and one does one's best to preserve this core value even in the midst of misfortune. As I sat in Casualty watching the calendar change, it occurred to me that wheels, and all that resembles them, are overdue for some serious reappraisal. The wheel is said to be the defining hallmark of civilisation, and, perhaps by extrapolation, cyclical thinking is becoming the defining mind-set of the professional intelligentsia. These days 'round is sound', as George Orwell might have sloganised. Well, I say a plague on all things circular. Call it post-traumatic stress if you like, but I maintain that the highways and side streets of British medical life have become dangerously

---

[5] Adapted from *Education for General Practice* (2001), **12**, 114–17.

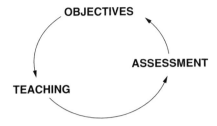

Figure 10.1   The Educational Paradigm.

congested with images of the wheel, and it's time some of them had a stick shoved in their spokes. You can't go very far in general practice these days without colliding with a cycle. An audit cycle, a budget cycle, an educational cycle, a decision-making cycle – there's always some smart-alecky model of the right way to do things; and that model is almost invariably wheel-shaped.

You know the sort of thing. Take the dear old Educational Paradigm, the three-stroke engine which allegedly powers vocational training (Figure 10.1). Your objectives determine your teaching, the effectiveness of which you submit to assessment, in order to set the next round of objectives.

Or the Audit Cycle (Figure 10.2). You pick on some defenceless aspect of performance. Measure it senseless. Hit it with a gold standard till it promises to do better. Sneak back later to see if it's pulled its socks up, and send it off round the course again if it hasn't.

Or the Budget Round (Figure 10.3), where you dream up a proposal that unfortunately will cost a bit, bid for funds, spend the money, account for it, make your excuses to the Treasurer, and come back with a revised bid or a revised proposal for the next financial year.

Circularity can infect Social Services too, if some of the meetings I've been to are any guide. They usually go like this. Adjusting our faces to a mask suitable of earnestness, we start by assessing the client's needs. Then we assign a key worker and allocate resources, and set up a review meeting to monitor the client's anticipated gratitude.

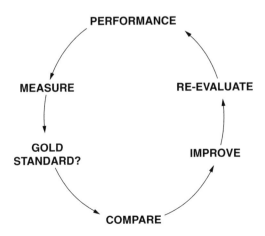

Figure 10.2   The Audit Cycle.

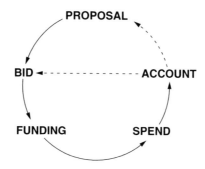

Figure 10.3   The Budget Round.

(This latter cycle has two common variants. In the first, after assessment of needs and allocation of resources comes down-sizing of resources, followed by setting up a review meeting on a date inconvenient for anyone who might not think the needs have actually been met. The other version goes: assess the needs, panic, share feelings of helplessness, decide the client didn't really understand what was needed in the first place.)

Underpinning all these examples is a belief that the only guarantee of effectiveness is a circular process based on a feedback loop, where the results of your actions endlessly come back to haunt you. Words like 'loop', 'cycle', 'round', 'paradigm' — they all seem able to invoke an awe to match that of stout Cortez on first beholding the Pacific Ocean. I'm sure you've all been at flipchart-littered seminars called something like 'Mousetraps for the New Millennium: towards a way forward'. Usually just before the afternoon tea break comes the 'insight moment' where the chief pundit, who has been charting the group discussion as it goes all round the houses, suddenly spots, to his great glee (and it always seems to be a 'he', doesn't it?), that an arrow can be drawn from the bottom of his flipchart right back up to the top of the page, thereby creating God's purest shape, the circle. Tea is taken in a mood of evangelical fervour, the eyes of the participants a-shining with Understanding, Vision and Purpose. Action planning for the future is polished off in twenty minutes flat and we all leave convinced that finally we have a model for achieving global mouselessness ...

... until, that is, it dawns on the way home that one's own part in the enterprise seems to consist mostly of counting an awful lot of dead mice.

Circular models of complex processes are attractive because they seem to give us an easy grip on slippery situations. They are all examples of a fundamental biological process, the feedback loop, designed to keep crucial variables from wandering too far off limits. Homeostasis, in a word. Eat a bar of chocolate, and the blood sugar rises. Some clever little 'spotter' cell notices, and gives the pancreatic islets a prod. On comes the insulin and back down goes the sugar level. Eat *sixteen* bars of chocolate, and some other clever little cell triggers the vomiting centre, and you won't do *that* again in a hurry. These are all circular processes, where output from the end stage is recycled as formative input for the first stage. Jolly clever. I should imagine Mother Nature must feel pretty smug about homeostasis.

When I got back to work I started to say as much to Greg. 'Yes,' he said, 'it's what I think you'll find mathematicians call an iterative process.' And before I could say 'Go on', he went on. 'The results of Round 1 become the starting point for Round 2, as with the Mandelbrot set of complex numbers c such that the repeated mapping $z \rightarrow z^2 + c$ converges to a finite value. Or,' he continued relentlessly, 'the way you convert ? to a decimal. 3s into 1 won't go; 3s into 10 goes 3, carry 1; 3s into 10 goes 3, carry 1; 3s into 10 − and so on until you get ...'

'Get bored?', I suggested. 'Or get close to slapping you in the face with a kipper?'

'No,' he replied, 'until you get to an acceptable approximation to some theoretically-ideal-but-never-quite-attained end point. Oh and by the way, we're out of biscuits.'

Back in the security of my professorial armchair I reflected that the result of cyclical activity, indeed its very purpose, is stability. Feedback loops bring a system to rest in a steady state which is sturdily resistant to outside influence. Circularity − not sowing unless you dare to reap, and sowing only what you have previously reaped − is the Conservatism of the natural world, protecting it from oscillation, perturbation and wobble. Circularity preserves the *status* very-nearly-*quo*. You work up a sweat, but go nowhere very fast.

As a concept, homeostasis may be all well and good where biological variables are concerned, but transposing it to the world of ideas and behaviour and education and development can be like putting sugar in the petrol tank. Wheel-shaped patterns of activity, like all circular processes, are only valid within closed systems. They lead us to believe that there is nothing of worth outside them, that there is no need for contact with, or input from, anything not already part of the little local universe. They foster the uniform at the expense of the inspired. They inhibit us from shedding the irrelevant, abandoning the futile and challenging the false assumption. They stifle initiative beneath endless analysis; they bind us to the treadmill and preclude the creative leap; they allow stagnant self-congratulation to flourish where a little self-questioning or self-stretching might be more apropos.

Iterative cyclical processes are great for fine-tuning − but only as long as you can safely assume that the right thing is being fine-tuned. The educational paradigm will ensure that all learning objectives are met − but only the ones you first thought of. Where do enthusiasm, curiosity, humanity or fun get a look in?

According to the clinical governance creed, we should be auditing much of what we do. Fair enough. But can the audit cycle tell us what it is in our own practice that needs attention? What next? Or what most urgently?

And in the eternal budget round, including at national level, is it really good enough to keep on redefining needs as no more than can be successfully bid for?

Part of the trouble is that the very words we associate with roundness have deeply ingrained positive vibes. The wheel of life; the wheel to which one's shoulder should be put; coming full circle or moving in the best ones; the cycles lunar, menstrual, Krebs and of Toscanini's Beethoven symphonies − all have connotations of prosaic mortals humbled in contemplation of natural rhythm and a Higher Power. But try saying instead 'educational treadmill', or 'audit tail-chase', or 'budget merry-go-round', and already you have a sense that the pedestal could crumble.

Faced with any problem-solving model that's starting to look prescriptively circular, I propose we ask ourselves a number of questions before it's too late.

- Will this approach lead us into an open or a closed system?
- If open, where will fresh input come from?
- If closed, what might be being excluded from it?
- How could we break out of the circle if we wanted to?
- How would we know whether we were trapped in the circle or not?

Musing thus, I must have fallen into another of those fitful professorial interludes which the casual passer-by might mistake for dozing. Images of circularity in action crowded in. In a nightmare vision of the future of general practice I saw the GP as a juggler in a circus ring, setting plates labelled diabetes, hypertension, appointment systems and epilepsy spinning on the canes of audit, dashing ever more desperately from plate to wobbling plate as the numbers grew unmanageable. 'Send in the clowns!' I longed to scream. There ought to be clowns. I dreamed of the legendary Woozalum bird, which flew around in such increasingly tight circles that it ended up beyond the help even of the finest proctologists in Harley Street. I recalled Kekule's self-ingesting snake, and was shuddering at doing so unsavoury a thing to one's own backside when Greg burst into the room, startling me back into semi-coherence.

'Nature', I exclaimed before he could speak, 'doesn't require her creations to consume their own droppings, does she? Waste matter returning to the environment makes a contribution – of course it does – to the vigour of the biosphere as a whole. But only as a general fertilizer, not as a tonic to the individual.'

Greg was looking at me strangely.

'Fine tuning killed the dinosaurs,' I prattled. 'The only good thing to go round and round is a mulberry bush. Wheels are for going places. If a wheel doesn't help you get somewhere fresh, get a horse. Or skis. Or a hovercraft. Sometimes it's good to wobble.'

'You're hysterical,' he said, and slapped me. 'Anyway, I've been giving some thought to the biscuit problem and I've come up with a protocol. Each morning I stock-take the biscuit tin and evaluate it against an agreed minimal contents threshold. If necessary, this triggers in-team fund-raising, thus empowering a Consultation and Acquisition Working Group with replenishment capability ...'

'Greg,' I said, feeling much restored, though for some reason still aware of the residual bruising from the impact with his bicycle, 'go buy some custard creams.'

And I bunged him a quid. There. Easy.

11

'Nothing either good or bad . . .'

What follows is a transcript of my Richard Scott Memorial Lecture, given in Edinburgh in June 2001.

Richard Scott, an Edinburgh GP and an energetic supporter of the Royal College of General Practitioners in its early years, was appointed in 1963 to the world's first Chair of General Practice, at Edinburgh University. The lecture that bears his name was inaugurated in 1989.

' . . . but thinking makes it so'[1]

In my limited experience, speakers on commemorative occasions such as this fall into one of four categories. Some will tell you about their latest research findings. Sadly my only piece of original research was done a long time ago when I was an undergraduate at Cambridge. It concerned the neuro-psychology of sleep, and proved that no matter how loud a noise you make in the proximity of sleeping medical students, some will always manage to sleep through it. Besides, whatever it is we need at the moment to enhance the vigour of primary care, journal-loads of new clinical facts aren't it.

A second group of lecturers will turn in an exquisitely witty after dinner speech, full of jokes and anecdotes about the funny things patients say. (Actually, I had a pregnant lady in last week, she hands me a urine sample, and says, 'Would you mind testing this, because last time the midwife said it had croutons in it.')

The third group are the visionaries – I'm thinking of people like my good friend Iona Heath – people for whom general practice allows a deep and privileged involvement with the all the joys and anguish and mystery of the human condition, and who can distil from that wonderful complexity an inspiration that reminds us that ours is a job supremely worth doing. Much of what we do is precious and subtle, yet at the same time vulnerable and easily misunderstood, and I yield to no one in my admiration of anyone who can articulate the unique value of our discipline. But you, I think, are not an audience who needs reminding of it. Indeed, there is a danger that *just* reminding ourselves – just reminding *ourselves* – of what we believe in risks a retreat into helpless nostalgia from which it is but a short step to extinction. The defining millennial image of general practice should not be a group of teary-eyed dinosaurs swapping tales of the good old days before the asteroid struck.

So a fourth category of people in my position will, like the bore there's usually one of at parties, regale you at length on the subjects of what's wrong with

---

[1] 'There is nothing either good or bad, but thinking makes it so.' Shakespeare: *Hamlet*, Act II, scene ii.

the world, and what needs doing about it. The culprits usually turn out to be the powers that be – managers, politicians, the usual suspects – and the solution is usually to slip something into the drinking water that will make everybody see things our way. To a 'here tonight, gone in the morning' speaker the role of Eeyore is an attractive one, and (I have to warn you) one I've not managed completely to resist. But I'll try to mix in elements of the first three categories – well, the visionary and the humorous ones, not the research. I'm going to offer some historical and philosophical perspectives on why it might be that many of us feel a deep unease, a distinct queasiness, about where general practice seems presently to be headed. I'll suggest that some, but not all, of the underlying pathology resides in some fallacies and wrong assumptions in the way we think about things, and a degree of foolishness in some of the ways we allow matters that concern us to be conducted. I'll be suggesting that, as a profession and possibly as a College, we're displaying a corporate naïvety about how things get decided and implemented in the real world. Inoffensive and genteel though we might wish to remain, *not* to evolve new behaviours and survival strategies during a period of political climate change risks betraying our visionary inheritance.

Anyway – let me tell you a story. It's a true story, and it will serve as a metaphor for my whole thesis.

Some years ago I was examining for the MRCGP Orals in Edinburgh. One day I shared a table with David Haslam, now the Chairman-Elect of Council but at that time still a mortal like the rest of us. In the morning we oralled a young doctor from the Western Highlands, who was excellent. He was knowledgeable, kind, thoughtful, enthusiastic, first class in every way. Then in the afternoon we had another doctor from the same town, older, clearly more senior, and very very Scots. 'Oh,' we said, 'another doctor from …' 'Aye,' he said, 'I think ya had ma trrrrainee this morrrning.' David asked him the following question. 'Suppose you received a letter from your local Consultant Radiologist telling you that, for some reason, he was having to withdraw from GPs the privilege of ordering barium X-rays – how would you deal with that?' 'It's no' a problem I would anticipate having,' came the reply. 'Why not?' says Haslam. 'I'm Chairman of the Boarrrrd.'

Now, David Haslam didn't get where he is today by being for long at a loss for words, so he persisted: 'OK, that's a string that only you can pull. If you couldn't pull that string, how would you deal with the situation?' There was the briefest pause, then the candidate, miming suitably, said, 'I'd lift the phone, I'd get through, I'd say, "Georrrrge, what the f**k?"'

At school I was never any good at history – at least, not the sort that means being able to recite the causes of the First World War. On the other hand I did have one inspirational teacher of Latin and Greek – Frank Thomas – who taught me to appreciate the merits of a civilisation based on Classical values. Frank also conducted the school orchestra, and, when I showed some ability on the violin, introduced me to the string quartet repertoire and in particular to the Romantic composers. 'Someone who doesn't like Schubert,' he would say, 'got no soul.' And, if I were so bold as to attempt to set an explanatory framework for the development of European civilisation, I should do so in terms of those twin traditions, the Classical and the Romantic. The history of our thought and philosophy, our art, our ideas, our political and civil institutions is the story of creative tension between the Classical and Romantic mind-sets.

The Classical frame of mind attempts to find order in the midst of chaos. It aspires to tame the natural wilderness. The Classical virtues are regularity, harmony, balance, rationality, objectivity, control. People of a Classical persuasion are attracted to logic, symmetry, rules, principles, guidelines, generalisations. Classicists are our natural law-*makers*. Romantics, on the other hand, are more interested in the individual's unique place in the world. Romanticism emphasises the subjective, the spontaneous, the imaginative, the irrational, the exceptional, the unpredictable and uninhibited. Romantics are our natural law-*breakers* – visionaries, subversives, iconoclasts. To a Classicist, the structure is the thing. 'By all means express your individuality,' says the Classicist, 'but within bounds.' To the Romantic, freedom is the thing. 'By all means let us have rules,' the Romantic replies, 'as long as they serve to emancipate and celebrate our diversity.'

And, from the alternation and interplay between these our two Janus faces, the achievements of our society continue to emerge. Over time, ascendancy passes from Classical to Romantic and back again. Cultures evolve much as species do. Romantic variation is acted on by the Classical forces of natural selection, and the fittest survive.

As an example, let's see if this idea of a Classical/Romantic split holds up in our own professional sphere, and take a retrospective glance at the history of general practice from 1200 BC to the present day. Very briefly: Aesculapius-style healing was part of magic, a question of propitiating the gods through ritual – highly Romantic. With Empedocles in the 5th century BC we find the first attempts to bring some Classical order to understanding disease, the aim of healthcare being to restore harmony between the four bodily humours: blood, phlegm, yellow and black bile. The Classical model reached its first flowering with Hippocrates, who insisted that disease was a natural rather than a supernatural phenomenon, and that we needed nothing more than the evidence of our senses and our reason to understand its causes and treatment.

In Western Europe, the authority of the Christian Church had an adverse effect upon medical progress. The human body was held sacred and dissection was forbidden. Disease was regarded as a punishment for sin, and treatment primarily a matter of prayer and repentance. In such an anti-intellectual Romantic climate, a Classical tradition stayed alive only with difficulty. Medicine before the Enlightenment must have felt very similar to our own present experience. The Classical spirit endowed the great Universities and schools of medicine. Vesalius, Harvey, Paré – all took their giant steps in the rational advancement of anatomy, physiology and surgery. And yet at the same time witchcraft and alchemy flourished, and members of the then new medical Royal Colleges pored over the contents of the chamber pot in a Romantic hope of finding a diagnosis in it.

With the Age of Enlightenment and the rise of scientism, the pendulum swung very firmly in the Classical direction, leading eventually to the enormous achievements of what we've come to refer to as the 'medical model', with its emphasis on logic, analysis, structure, authority and evidence. Yet, as we know, it wasn't long before we general practitioners were itching for a Romantic backlash against the Classical rigidities of the medical model, carving out our own territory in which we could feel at ease with such wobbly and (to a Classicist) self-indulgent notions as 'the management of uncertainty', or 'the doctor-patient relationship', 'the doctor as drug', 'the apostolic function', and 'the art of general practice'.

Even within the recent history of our own discipline we can see the tension between Classicism and Romanticism creatively at work. As an example of the hybrid vigour that can arise when Classical and Romantic values are allowed to cross-pollinate, I'd cite that seminal work of the 1970s, *The future general practitioner*. That book was conceived when general practice was searching Romantically for self-importance and climbed into bed with Classical educational theory, an encounter that has generated thirty years of energy in vocational training. Another example – all those models of the consultation that delight some people and irritate others are fusions between Romantic visions of what matters and a Classical belief that things ought to make sense. And all those poor Registrars whose consultations I and my fellow examiners for the MRCGP watch on video are clearly struggling to impose some Classical rigour on their own unstructured and Romantic ideas of what consulting is about. What's more, having written highly Romantic books about the relationships between doctors and patients, or trainers and registrars, I was once accused of hypocrisy at an MRCGP exam preparation course by a candidate who thought that this didn't square with a Classical exam which is all about standards and reliability and validity and statistics and regula-tions. Touché, I thought – except that it doesn't *feel* like hypocrisy. To a Gemini like me, it *feels* OK to have a foot in both camps, to espouse *both* sets of values without having to deny either, to like cheese *and* pudding.

I don't imagine I'm alone in this, am I? Isn't it perfectly acceptable – healthy, even – to spend Tuesday afternoon Classically auditing one's management of hypertension, then on the Wednesday go off Romantically to one's Balint group?

The point is, it's possible for the pull between these two tendencies to enlarge us rather than distort us: to stretch us gently so that we grow, rather than violently so that we break.

A positive outcome *is* possible – but it's not guaranteed. Which brings me, perhaps laboriously, to attempt a diagnosis of that professional unease I spoke of about what's happening to general practice at the moment, that queasy feeling many of us have that we GPs are perched precariously like Humpty-Dumpty on a high wall, eyeing rather nervously all the hob-nailed boots and trampling hooves of the men and horses beneath us.

The way I read it, the natural state of general practice (left to our own devices) is at the present time significantly Romantic. I think – for all that we willingly accept the need for accountability and quality control and evidence-base and consistency and other hallmarks of a Classical value-system – we are not yet ready to turn our backs on Romantic views of what it means to be personal doctors. To us Romantics, the guidelines and targets and algorithms beloved of the Classical theorists are to our preferred way working pretty much what pebbles on the beach are to the would-be bather. We want still to be able to take constructive delight in the unique stories of individual patients. We want still to be bespoke tailors, cutting the cloth of health care to fit the ungainly bulges of individual patients in ways that off-the-peg garments, no matter how smart, may not do[2].

Our difficulty is, we find ourselves at present in a political context where Classical values of a rather aggressive kind are in the ascendancy. But it is not a

---

[2] Reviewing this text for publication only three years later, but in a post-New Contract world with its Quality and Outcomes Framework, I have to say it looks as if the pendulum has started its swing away from Romanticism earlier than I had expected.

Classical context that feels sure enough of its merits to dare to clasp the Romantic tendency in creative embrace. Seemingly laudable slogans such as 'levelling up', 'combating inequality' and 'a new beginning' are frequently camouflage for some rather spiteful and disreputable creatures – an abrogation of central responsibilities, a fear of local initiative, a top-down bullying approach to agenda-setting.

It's not hard to see why this is – indeed, I suspect 'twas ever thus. As Machiavelli was brave enough to acknowledge, politics is principally about gaining and retaining power. There's nothing dishonourable about that in itself; but all kinds of foolishness can arise when we – governors and governed alike – collude in pretending that anything else is the case.

That politics is about power is the first of its two main axioms. The second axiom of politics – indeed, of life itself – is that delivery always falls short of expectation. People always want more than can be provided. It follows inevitably that dissatisfaction is endemic in the system, and that disappointment, sooner or later, is the end result of all political activity. Politics – the art of the possible – is therefore the art of managing disappointment. As far as I can see, every piece of political agenda goes through three stages, designed to manage disappointment, or at least to stave off disappointment long enough for power to be retained regardless.

The three stages of the political process in a democracy are – Promise, Pretend, Blame. You begin by promising enough to gain power. As the early signs of disappointment begin to appear, you pretend things are better than they are. When finally it becomes impossible to pretend that promises are being kept or expectations fulfilled, you distance yourself from responsibility, usually by identifying an enemy or scapegoat who can shoulder the blame, and whom you promise to tackle in the next round of the political cycle. Promising 'a better Health Service' gets you elected. Before long, however, you find yourself having to pretend that what you meant by 'better' wasn't faster treatment but more treatment episodes. By 'better access to primary care' you meant NHS Direct, not more GPs. By 'shorter waiting lists', you didn't actually mean to count people waiting to go on to the waiting list. When you spoke of raising clinical standards, you didn't mean a coordinated programme of educational opportunities for doctors – you meant orchestrating public indignation whenever there's an outrage such as Harold Shipman or a Bristol heart scandal. So who's to blame? Not the Government, squire – they've thrown money at the NHS, laid down frameworks, ordained national plans, set up advisory bodies, published statistics, defined targets, created Primary Care Trusts, all fully in accordance with the Classical notions of how disorder is to be regulated.

As an example of the 'promise/pretend/blame cycle' in operation, look at how the issue of access to the new but expensive treatments for neurological diseases (such as beta-interferon for multiple sclerosis) has been managed. An electorate constantly told that the NHS is the envy of the world reads in its newspapers of the latest wonder drug and, not unreasonably, assumes that a treatment that looks promising is a treatment that has been promised. When, funds being as short as they are, the inevitable postcode lottery develops, the Department of Health slips into 'pretend and blame' mode. 'The problem isn't shortage of money, and there need be no postcode lottery,' it asserts. 'What's lacking is clinical evaluation, which is the responsibility of the National Institute for Clinical Excellence'. Unfortunately NICE has been seduced into playing the promise/pretend/blame game as well.

It promised an independent appraisal of beta-interferon, but quickly had to pretend that in many cases the lack of firm evidence *for* effectiveness was the same as firm evidence *against* it. The upshot was a set of arbitrary guidelines which are scientifically unsound and, in human terms, deeply distressing for individual patients and clinicians. Yet it is those individual patients and clinicians who are left holding the blame for the present unsatisfactory situation on the grounds that they won't accept the guidelines!

Or – another example – out-patient waiting lists. Government, quite rightly, recognises that they are far too long for what claims to be a civilised society, and is elected on a promise to cut them. From Richmond House this instruction trickles down to individual hospitals and consultants, who find, since illness does not vanish simply because it's inconvenient and since they have no additional resources with which to tackle it, that the waiting lists remain deaf to political rhetoric. So what happens? Statistics are massaged and the definition of 'being on a waiting list' is adjusted so that, for a while, the pretence of improvement can be sustained. But now what do I read on the front page of the newspaper[3]? 'One in four GP referrals "wrong"'. Apparently the National Audit Office has published a report based on a questionnaire survey of consultants, who deem 25% of the out-patient referrals 'inappropriate', as a result of which they will not be able to 'meet their waiting list targets'. What cheek! 'Inappropriate' by whose lights? The Department of Health's? The Primary Care Organisation's? Probably not the consultants' – at least, not if they keep their clinical hats on. Probably not the GPs', who know all the underlying and complex reasons for making referrals. And certainly not the patients'. But promise has turned to pretence, and pretence to blame, and blame has been passed as far away from the centre as it's possible to get in the NHS – to general practice.

I think – (and I am trying to rise above the morass of local stupidities and to keep sight of the bigger picture) – I do think general practice is a largely Romantic profession struggling at the moment to find a best fit within a resolutely Classical political establishment – and not making a very good fist of it.

The value systems of general practice and political authority seem to be currently out of synch. And the cause of delivering good health care is suffering as a result. I think there's copious evidence that this is the case. The first casualty in any conflict of ideas is rational thought. If we look at some of the ways of thinking that we're starting to take for granted, some of our assumptions about how things can be made to improve, it seems to me that common sense has been grievously wounded.

Take how we think about change.

Probably the best form of change starts with a good idea from the bottom of the power pyramid and bubbles its way up, being refined and clarified as it rises. But, as we know to our cost, it's much more likely to start with a diktat at the top and become more and more complicated and unwieldy as it sinks ever lower. In a 'top down' power pyramid, it seems that all a suggestion has to be is plausible and novel for it to become imposed policy. The trouble is, human beings are capable of generating ideas much faster than they can be appraised, let alone implemented. The result is such a proliferation of so-called improvements that we at the grass roots can't keep track of them, let alone take them to our bosoms. The only thing that seems immune to endless innovation is the system that imposes it. As James

---

[3] *Daily Telegraph*, Wednesday June 6th 2001.

Willis says in his recent book *Friends in low places*[4], 'A thousand good ideas add up to a bureaucratic nightmare.' He's a sound chap, this Willis. I quote him again:

> 'When you examine what people who urge us to welcome change ... are actually saying, you nearly always find they are promoting *their* change. They want *us* to move quickly to do what ... *they* want ... It is often forgotten that one of the adverse side-effects of (imposed) change is that it is profoundly inhibitory to personally directed change and therefore profoundly damaging to motivation.'

Government absolutely has the right to identify problems, and to demand that they be tackled. But if Government imposes a fresh solution on every problem it can think of, or if it starts to believe it has a monopoly on how solutions are devised and implemented, the resulting loss of motivation and goodwill amongst those of us who have to implement them may be catastrophic. In seeking to be tough on quality, our political masters are too tough on the *causes* of quality. *Enforcing* improvement is the greatest obstacle to securing it.

I'm sure we all have a story to tell of nonsense being perpetrated in the name of quality improvement. Perhaps you get slapped on the wrist by your prescribing advisor because you've committed the cardinal sin of prescribing something that wasn't fully evidence-based; or slapped on the other wrist by your clinical governance lead for not prescribing something expensive that was. Perhaps you've been seduced into participating in a Primary Care Organisation on the grounds that 'local control of resources' is a good thing, only to discover that doctor has been set against doctor to squabble over inadequacies not of their making and which they are powerless to rectify.

Does speaking in this way make me a cynic? I do hope so. A cynic – and you can quote me – a cynic is just a coward trying to look brave. I'll willingly put my hand up to cowardice, because picking these kinds of bones with the powers that be isn't what I joined the profession for, and it scares me. But trying to look brave is the first step to actually getting braver, and that's what I think it's time we did – got braver.

What does it mean, that attempt at a rallying cry – 'It's time for general practice to get braver'?

In the terms I've used in this address, it means protecting and advocating the Romantic streak in our values, so that it can contribute fully to the next stage of evolution of the nation's healthcare systems. It means not conceding that our core values are just vacuous froth that can be sacrificed to short-term political expediency, and that can be bullied out of the way if they conflict with Government's need for quick fixes. For general practice to get braver does not require the victory of Romantic medicine over Classical, nor vice versa, as if the two were doomed forever to be in conflict. It means rather arranging a marriage between them, insisting that they make love not war. It means being proud that general practice is one of the few remaining repositories in professional life of broad-band human values, and accepting the responsibility that places on us to be their champion.

The task *ought* to be – *can* be – easy. It means saying 'no' to what frustrates excellence, and 'yes' to what fosters it, regardless of the consequences. It means

---

[4] Willis J (2001) *Friends in low places*. Radcliffe Medical Press, Oxford.

denouncing the Classical fallacy that a stream of small short-term reforms inevitably build into substantial long-term progress. It means not being bounced into accepting endless imposed top-down idiocies, where all a suggestion need be is plausible for it to be promoted as 'good practice'. It means, if necessary, arguing against the array of regulatory mechanisms which have been imposed on us, such as Primary Care Organisations, the Commission for Health Improvement, National Service Frameworks – even if necessary against programmes of clinical appraisal and revalidation – if these developments serve primarily to distance Central government from the shortcomings of its own policy and provision.

'Being braver' means challenging some basic assumptions. Alan Milburn[5] said on the radio on May 22nd 2001, 'The only way to improve the NHS is to continue the programme of reform.' No, it isn't the only way. Reform ought to flow from proper thought, good ideas, and the abandonment of vested interest, and when this has not been the case we need the courage to say so.

However, it is not enough for the views of those of us at the bottom of the power pyramid to be logical, sensible, compassionate, constructive, radical, widely-held and well-expressed. To be persuasive to the political decision-makers at the top of the pyramid, our views also have to be safe – or at least, safer than theirs. And since to a politician safe means popular with the electorate, whatever case we want to advance has to command greater public support than theirs. In other words, our task is largely an educational one, to mobilise public understanding of what is at stake. And education is something that we as doctors and as members of this Royal College of General Practitioners ought to be good at.

As a profession, our daily stock in trade is our understanding of how human beings function – what worries them, what motivates them, what they expect and how they learn. We have creativity in abundance, massive public esteem, and, for Heaven's sake, we have communication skills. We also, in the form of the College, have an organisation. Surely we ought to be able to harness all these resources in pursuit of something better than our present wing-and-a-prayer health service? Just as we GPs act as advocates for our patients, championing their individual causes and working to achieve the best possible congruence between the needs of the individual and the constraints of the system, so we as a profession should look to our College for just such advocacy on our own behalf. I should like to see the College undertaking a major and high profile programme to raise the big questions about health and health care on a massive public scale. I'd like to see the College as a showcase for big ideas. The College has the skills, the people and the resources to organise national debate on the big questions, such as, 'What is health? To what extent is it the individual's or the state's responsibility? What standards are we willing to pay for? How does health care here stand in comparison with other countries? What is the right balance between high tech. and low tech. treatments? How seriously should we take health inequalities?'

At the bottom of every sheet of College headed notepaper, in quite small print, is its mission statement, 'Promoting excellence in family medicine'. Promoting? What is the use of just 'promoting'? We should be 'demanding' excellence on behalf of the patients we serve, yelling our heads off about it! As the procession of the new NHS rolls past, and a ticker-tape blizzard of white papers, guidelines and

---

[5] Then the Secretary of State for Health.

manifestos cascades down from on high, the College should be that child in the crowd calling out, 'The Emperor has no clothes!'

I'm aware that, to a College whose temperament inclines more towards conciliation than confrontation, this will sound dangerously close to sedition. Saying 'no' to tyranny is a high-risk strategy, especially when the tyrant carries a captured banner emblazoned 'The Public Good'. But can we afford *not* to venture it? One of the College's pressing problems is retaining its membership. The MRCGP delivers about 1500 potential new paying members each year, but a good many each year fail to renew. I suspect that many lapsed members feel the College has failed to stand for big enough things, or to stand firmly enough against the big dangers. I would urge us all to learn from the example of another Romantic who found himself struggling to retain human values as the world lurched, for all the right reasons, towards the catastrophe of World War – E M Forster. In a magnificent essay called 'What I believe', Forster wrote as follows.

> 'One must be fond of people and trust them if one is not to make a mess of life, and it is therefore essential that they should not let one down. They often do. The moral of which is that I must, myself, be as reliable as possible. But reliability is not a matter of contract – that is the main difference between the world of personal relationships and the world of business relationships. It is a matter for the heart, which signs no documents ... Personal relationships are despised today. They are regarded as bourgeois luxuries, as products of a time of fair weather which is now past, and we are urged to get rid of them, and to dedicate ourselves to some movement or cause instead. I hate the idea of causes, and if I had to choose between betraying my country and betraying my friend, I hope I should have the guts to betray my country ... Love and loyalty to an individual can run counter to the claims of the State. When they do – down with the State, say I.'

I knew Forster slightly when I was an undergraduate. He was a modest man, self-effacing, and I have some small sense of what a brave thing it would have been for him to express so seditious an idea. But there are thousands of us, and it's not actually war towards which we are lurching. I should like the defining image of millennial general practice to be not the nostalgic dinosaurs, but Socrates – that irascible and rascally maverick of Classical Athens. Every day Socrates would take his place in the main square in full view of the seat of civic power, and would draw the great and the good of his day into reluctant debate, forcing them through remorseless questioning to confront the shoddy basis in philosophy for their all-too-easy assumptions, until some humility in the face of life's interconnectedness penetrated their smart-aleck minds.

So I for one am with that second doctor from the Western Highlands, and I hope that if – *when* – we have to choose between serving our patient and serving our political masters we shall have the guts to say, 'Georrrge,' (or, as it might be, Tony, or Michael) 'what the ... ?'

12

The little mushroom and the blighted twin

In 1981 the then *Journal of the Royal College of General Practitioners* published, as an 'individual study', a paper of mine entitled 'Antenatal memories and psychopathology'[1]. This was its summary:

> 'A case is described of suicidal impulses apparently stemming from the patient's experience before and during his birth. By using a technique of "rebirthing", antenatal memories were relived and their traumatic effects resolved. Theoretical and practical accounts of rebirthing are given, and its significance for general practitioners is discussed.'

There is abundant evidence in the psychological literature of the personality-shaping and vulnerability-determining effects of intrauterine life. Over the course of my professional career I've done birth regression work, or made productive pregnancy-related interpretations, with perhaps a dozen individuals, usually at times of life crisis.

We in general practice are used to making diagnoses in physical, psychological and social terms. My early paper proposed a fourth category, diagnosis in metaphorical terms, to remind us to wonder, 'What meaning does this illness, or these symptoms, have for the individual?' The metaphorical aspect of disease is implicit when we ask, for example, the neurodermatitis sufferer what has got under her skin, or the dyspeptic whom he is sick of, or the agoraphobic what relationship she feels trapped by. Spotting the metaphor can give insight into the time and circumstances when a patient failed to cope with some trauma or stress.

I went on to suggest that an important feature of intuitive medicine was the ability to make metaphorical 'as if' hypotheses, connecting patterns and themes in a patient's behaviour and feelings with some model of human development, which might include intrauterine development. Stanislav Grof[2] and Frank Lake[3] went further, describing how the connections might be more than metaphor, and in fact represent transforms of memories of actual prenatal and perinatal events. Grof's 'basic perinatal matrices' offer a physiologically-based framework for interpreting many symptom clusters and behaviours as birth metaphors. The 'feel' of situations and relationships one keeps getting 'into' may recapture qualities of that primal

---

[1] *J. Roy. Coll. Gen. Pract.*, 1981, **31**, 751–5.
[2] Grof S (1975) *Realms of the human unconscious*. Viking Press, New York.
[3] Lake F (1979) The significance of perinatal experience. In *Birth and rebirth: self and society*. Special issue, June 1979, pp. 8–16. Bourne Press, London.

context, the womb[4]. Inexplicable feelings and reactions under stress and conflict, for example, may arise from emotional and physical memories of the events of labour and delivery.

One of my musical heroes since boyhood has been Franz Schubert (*see* Chapter 3, page 14), and one of my greatest passions has been his music. At some point I made the connection between various unexplained features of Schubert's life and works and what I had come to understand about foetal memory. The hypothesis suggested itself that Schubert may have been the singleton survivor of a 'blighted twin' pregnancy.

I presented this theory in an illustrated talk to a meeting at the Royal Society of Medicine over a decade ago. Something alarmingly close to fisticuffs broke out. Some of the audience said it was the biggest load of hogwash masquerading as science they had ever heard. Nonsense, riposted others, it was the most refreshing and original talk it had ever been their privilege … Friend berated friend, husband argued with wife. I slipped away in the confusion. Clearly, even the very possibility had touched some deep psychological strata.

But the idea didn't go away. In June 2000 I presented my thesis to an international conference organised by the Schubert Institute (UK) at the University of Leeds. Amongst musicians and musicologists, (not my usual audience), the 'blighted twin' hypothesis went down rather better. An expanded version was later published as a chapter in 'the book of the conference'[5], and is reproduced here by kind permission of the publishers and the editor, Professor Brian Newbould, to whom I am extremely grateful.

The Doppelgänger revealed?

Conscious that this paper will be read by professional musicians, musicologists and Schubert scholars, I should at once confess myself to be, in this company, an amateur. I'm a medical doctor, a general practitioner, with a special interest in psychotherapy, which means I'm especially curious about what makes people tick. A large part of my working life is spent wondering how individuals get to be the way they are, tracing the complexities of their present lives back to their origins in earlier, sometimes *much* earlier, formative experiences. A large part of my recreational life, on the other hand, has been spent in the company of Franz Schubert. As a lifelong violinist, and thanks to an early introduction to playing his symphonies and chamber works, I'm passionate about Schubert, and – not surprisingly in view of my professional background – I'm particularly interested in how he and his music might have got to be the way they are.

I shall begin by posing some unsolved conundrums about Schubert's life, personality and music. Then I shall describe how, in general terms, such conundrums sometimes can be answered in terms of very early experience – even as early as the life of the unborn baby in the womb. Finally I shall speculate that, in Schubert's case, for him to have undergone one particular such prenatal experience might account for some aspects of his life and work that we find puzzling.

---

[4] Laing RD (1976) *The facts of life*. Allen Lane, London.
[5] In Newbould B (ed.) (2003) *Schubert the progressive: history, performance practice, analysis*. Ashgate, Aldershot, pp. 139–49.

Conundrums

The better I become acquainted with Schubert's life and music, the more I find myself asking a number of questions to which the published canon of literature provides no plausible answers:

- Why was Schubert so particularly short in stature?
- How did he attain his emotional profundity?
- Why is a dactyl rhythm so common in his music?
- What are we to make of Schubert's 'volcanic outbursts'?
- What underlies the recurring pattern of his friendships?
- What was his attitude to death?

To elaborate briefly on each of these in turn:

Schubert's short stature

Schubert was very short, as Schober's well-known caricature of Schubert and Vogl illustrates and his nickname 'Schwammerl' – 'little mushroom' – confirms. When assessed for army conscription in 1818, his height was recorded as 4 feet, 11½ inches, and he was described as 'weak ... totally unserviceable'[6]. As far as we know, Schubert's parents were not particularly short. His brother Karl was described on the same occasion as 'tall', and his brother Ignaz, despite being hunch-backed, was about 5'6".

His emotional profundity

Listening to his music, we sense in Schubert a man emotionally wise way beyond his years. It might be said that, whereas with Mozart at his best we scale the heights and come down again, when Schubert is at his best we can plumb the soul's absolute depths and come up again. It is as if, as a youth, Schubert had already somehow acquired a mature personal familiarity with love, companionship, loneliness, despair and death, awaiting only a sufficient mastery of music's technicalities to give them expression in melody, rhythm and form. But the events and circumstances of his life always seem simply too ordinary to carry the weight of explanation for so seemingly innate and precocious a grasp of emotional complexity. None of the clichés of the lovesick artist starving in a garret apply to Schubert. He never went hungry, was never penniless, never wanted for company. Even his supposed infatuation with Therese Grob seems to have been altogether too light-weight an affair to have sensitised him so exquisitely and poignantly to the human condition. As the Viennese lawyer Heinrich Kreissle von Hellborn wrote in 1865,

> 'Schubert is, perhaps, a single instance of a great artist whose outer life had no affinity or connection with his art. His career was so simple and uneventful, so out of proportion with works that he created like a heavensent genius.'[7]

---

[6] Deutsch O, trans. Blom E (1946) *Schubert – a documentary biography*. J M Dent, London, p. 113.
[7] Quoted in Gibbs C (2000) *The life of Schubert*. Cambridge University Press, Cambridge, p. 6.

Schubert's dactyl rhythm

A 'long, short-short, long short-short' dactylic rhythm could be said to be Schubert's 'signature rhythm', occurring innumerable times throughout his oeuvre and from all stages of his composing career. The dactyl can be a slow 'minim and two crotchets', as for example in the 1817 song 'Der Tod und das Mädchen' (D. 531), or its 1824 transcription in the slow movement of the *String quartet in D minor* (D. 810). It can be a faster 'crotchet and two quavers' as in the *Wanderer fantasia* of 1822 (D. 760), or a quaver and two semi-quavers, as in 'Liebesbotschaft' from *Schwanengesang* (1828, D. 957). Schubert often combines the dactyl at two speeds, a fast version encompassed within half of a slower one, as for example in the *andante* of the 1824 *String quartet in A minor* (D. 804).

It seems likely, from the diversity and emotional range of the music that is pervaded with this rhythm, that a dactylic 'slow, quick-quick slow, quick-quick' was often for Schubert *le rhythme juste* – a personal rhythm that so often 'just felt right', one to which he returned time and again as to a favourite armchair[8]. Why might that be? Dietrich Fischer-Dieskau, in his book *Schubert: a biographical study of his songs*, asserts that the dactyl is,

> 'that secret heartbeat which accompanies the tread of death, and by means of which Schubert expresses that serenity which is death's alone.'[9]

Possibly dissatisfied with his own explanation, Fischer-Dieskau further speculates that the dactyl rhythm might represent,

> 'a secret argument as in the Chinese Book of Changes, in which one long dash signifies "Yes" and two short "No", (as is also) found in twelfth-century Japanese Gagaku-music.'[10]

That being as it may, there are many occasions where even the 'dactyl as symbol of death' idea simply does not fit the sense and feel of the music or (in the case of songs) the words. The dactyl seems always to be there as a kind of rhythmic origin to which Schubert frequently returns.

'Volcanic outbursts'

Hugh Macdonald coined this phrase in an article in the *Musical Times* entitled 'Schubert's Volcanic Temper'. In it he writes,

> 'In Schubert's instrumental music there is to be observed a phenomenon best described as his "volcanic temper" since it bears a striking resemblance to the two natural phenomena of volcanic eruption and of choleric temper. It represents a side of his art remote from the familiar lyrical Schubert ... There is a streak of violence and distemper in the music which makes itself known in unmistakeable ways.'[11]

---

[8] The late Philip Radcliffe, personal communication, c. 1990.
[9] Fischer-Dieskau D (1976) *Schubert: a biographical study of his songs.* Cassell, London. p. 85.
[10] *Op. cit.,* p. 85.
[11] Macdonald H (1978) Schubert's Volcanic Temper. *Musical Times*, vol. cxix, p. 949.

Examples include the almost panicky vocal entry after the lugubrious slow opening piano dactyls in the song 'Der Tod und das Mädchen'; the fortissimo interlude in the slow movement of the late *Piano sonata in A minor* (D. 959); and the terrifying passage towards the end of the 2nd movement of the *Symphony no. 9 in C major* (D. 944, bars 226–249), a movement also underpinned by an insistent dactyl rhythm.

Macdonald considers, only to dismiss, a number of theories as to the origin of such passages, finding no evidence of violence in Schubert's own personality as documented by his friends, nor of any musical need for the music to become violently disrupted. It appears that, rarely but inexplicably, Schubert felt impelled to create in music the effect of a cataclysmic dislocation of what had hitherto been tranquil.

Schubert's friendships

For much of his life Schubert shared confidences and lodgings with a succession of male friends, such as Mayrhofer, Senn and Schober. I neither wish nor need to enter the debate concerning the sexual proclivities of Schubert and his circle[12]. Some were possibly homosexual, others not. But at any given moment there always to seems to have been one particular person with whom Schubert was currently 'best friends' and from whom he was, at least temporarily, inseparable. Whether by accident or design (and in matters of subconscious motivation very few things are thought to happen by accident), most of these close relationships either proved transient or ended in betrayal and disappointment. Conventional psychoanalytic thought, faced with repetitive and compulsive behaviour of this kind, would seek an explanation in terms of infantile or pre-infantile experience.

Schubert's attitude to death

Schubert had a lifelong presentiment that he would die young. In the poems about death which he chose for his song settings, death is seen as a welcome release from anguish, something warm, comforting, and almost maternal. While this was indeed a common view of Romantic poets at the time, nevertheless Schubert seems, as a moth to a candle, to have been particularly attracted to it. Not only in *Winterreise* (D. 910) does the composer seem to identify with the role of the wanderer, roaming alone and bereft through a hostile environment until death brings his loneliness to a longed-for end. *Sehnsucht* ('longing'), arguably an over-worked idea in the poetic vocabulary of Schubert's time, seems to feature unusually prominently in the texts he chose to set to music, and to carry the particular connotation of a longing for death.

Fischer-Dieskau observes, quoting eighteen *lieder* as examples, that Schubert,

> 'the artist, did *not* long for death, (if by that we mean) the dark side of life. It is
> indeed remarkable how seldom the songs that deal with death leave the

[12] See, for example, Solomon M (1989) 'Franz Schubert and the Peacocks of Benvenuto Cellini'. *19th-Century Music*, vol. xii/3, pp. 193–206.

listener with a feeling of sadness. The central experience of such songs is rather one of consolation and trustful optimism.'[13]

In spite of an almost morbid preoccupation with death, Schubert does not appear, from the testimony of his friends, to have suffered from what we should now call depression. The attractiveness of death does not seem to represent an active impulse to suicide; rather is it an impatience to find a remedy for separation and alienation which are his lot in the living world.

A hypothesis

Contemporary portraits of Schubert all show a face with a prominent forehead and with eyes, nose and mouth relatively close to each other, occupying a slightly smaller than usual proportion of the head. This, together with his short stature, suggest to my medical eye that Schubert was affected by something called 'intra-uterine growth retardation' (IUGR). This means that while he was still an unborn baby in his mother Elizabeth's womb something had stunted his growth. Babies to whom this happens are often small as adults – smaller than the heights of their parents would lead one to expect – and with features similar to those Schubert is depicted as possessing. Medical conditions which can cause IUGR include:

• Serious illness or malnutrition in the mother
• Threatened miscarriage
• Infarction (partial death) of the placenta
• Congenital abnormality affecting the baby
• Infections, e.g. German measles
• A twin or triplet pregnancy
• 'Blighted twin' pregnancy.

The last condition listed, 'blighted twin' pregnancy, is interesting. Approximately one pregnancy in 80 results in the birth of twins. Occasionally, however, one of twin foetuses may for a variety of reasons die at some stage during the pregnancy, leaving the surviving twin to continue developing and ultimately to be born as a single baby. Particularly in the case of identical twins, who share a single placenta, the survivor may be affected with IUGR and exhibit the small stature and facial features associated with this condition.

Now suppose – just suppose – that the one twin destined to survive realised (whatever that means) what was happening as its sibling perished. Suppose that, in some sense as yet to be determined, it knew that it once had 'another half' in the womb who, inexplicably, no longer existed. What might be the effects of that awareness on the survivor?

It may startle you to know, as indeed once it startled *me*, that this notion of 'foetal memory' is more than speculation. There is now abundant evidence from clinical psychologists and therapists that some of these very early pre-natal experiences are in some form 'remembered', and that they exert profound influences over the psychological make-up of the adult whom that foetus will eventually become.

---

[13] *Op. cit.*, p. 207.

Intra-uterine events are not remembered in specific visual images or words. But – if to remember means to be affected by the past – they are remembered nevertheless. They are perpetuated in the form of personality traits, as determinants of prevailing moods and attitudes; they are remembered in dreams, in behaviour patterns under stress, in aspirations and vulnerabilities. People are shaped – not exclusively, not inevitably, but nevertheless in some fundamental ways are shaped – by the things that happen to them before they are born. Some of these very early life events come to act as templates, moulds, for our personalities, shaping the way we shall in time come to view the world we are born into and the particular configurations of relationships we are able to form.

How might this be?

The early work on foetal memory goes back to Arthur Janov[14] and R D Laing[15] in the 1970s and 80s. Other researchers such as Grof[16], Feher[17] and Emerson[18] in the USA and Frank Lake[19,20] in the UK developed therapeutic techniques for recalling an awareness of intra-uterine life in adult patients. I myself published in 1981 an account of one particular case in which an inexplicably suicidal young man was enabled, through regression techniques, to relive and thereby discharge the distress with which he had been overwhelmed when, as a foetus of about 20 weeks gestation, he had been flooded with adrenalin when his mother was involved in a 'near miss' road accident[21].

We should not be surprised that the nervous system of a developing embryo is capable, within the limits of its physiological maturity, of reacting to events and stimuli in much the same way as it will do once beyond the arbitrary landmark of birth. Recent advances in neurophysiology (the science of how the brain works) show that the unborn baby even from about twelve weeks into the pregnancy has a brain already capable of doing what brains do – sleeping and waking, reacting to sensations and sounds, dreaming, responding to a wide range of hormones and chemicals called neurotransmitters – in a word, learning about, and being shaped by, the world it finds itself in. People are shaped – not exclusively, not inevitably, but nevertheless in some fundamental ways – by the things that happen to them before they are born[22].

It appears that there are at least two processes involved in human memory and learning, a 'fast track' and a 'slow track'. The fast track memory system is the more familiar one, based on electrical activity in the network of nerve cells that makes up the brain, and set in motion by information from our primary senses of sight, hearing and touch. This is the system that remembers, for instance, your home telephone number or your usual fingering for the tricky first violin passages in Schubert's *Quartett-Satz in C minor*. The slow track memory system is in many ways more interesting. It appears that some kinds of memory are mediated by

[14] Janov A (1983) *Imprints – the lifelong effects of the birth experience.* Coward-McCann, New York.

[15] Laing RD (1982) *The voice of experience.* Allen Lane, London.

[16] Grof S (1975) *Realms of the human unconscious.* Souvenir Press, London.

[17] Feher L (1980) *The psychology of birth.* Souvenir Press, London.

[18] Emerson W (1978) Life, birth and rebirth. *Eur. J. Human. Psychol.,* **vi**, no. 7, 17–22.

[19] Lake F (1982) *With respect.* Darton Longman & Todd, London.

[20] Lake F (c.1982) *Studies in constricted confusion – exploration of a pre- and peri-natal paradigm.* Privately circulated.

[21] Neighbour R (1981) Antenatal memories and psychopathology. *J. Roy. Coll. Gen. Pract.,* **31**, 751–5.

[22] See, for example, Rossi E (1986) *The psychobiology of mind-body healing.* Norton, New York.

chemical patterns in the brain rather than electrical ones. The fluid which bathes the cells of the brain is perfused by a subtly changing array of chemical substances whose effect is to predispose some general configurations of response in preference to others. This is the kind of memory which makes us feel happy in certain environments and sad in others, or find some situations stressful and others uplifting.

So let us consider the specific phenomenon of the 'blighted twin'.

From the survivor's point of view, you are of course completely unaware as yet of a life outside the womb. You see nothing, hear little, and feel only the grosser movements your mother makes. But, as a twin, you probably register the presence of someone else alongside you, someone whose presence you have always known and which you take for granted. Imagine that that someone suddenly perishes, possibly in some distress. As this physiological catastrophe unfolds, a rush of powerful hormones and other emotionally-active chemicals courses through your bloodstream, soaking into your brain and changing forever the architecture of your own developing psychological make-up. Your *alter ego*, your Doppelgänger, is gone. The two of you have been reduced to one – and yet that one remembers that being two was its original and natural condition.

So my hypothesis is that this is what may have happened to Schubert. I think Schubert experienced intra-uterine growth retardation. I think in Schubert we could have a man who was the singleton survivor of a twin pregnancy, the other half of which was blighted. I think we have a man who began life as one of a pair, and who, in mid-pregnancy, lay helplessly by while a twin sibling perished, while what was two was reduced to one. We have a man whose creative imagination was thereby predisposed to express an abiding sense of loss and incompleteness, in whose music we can discern an intra-uterine memory of an inseparable two becoming a bereft and forlorn one. We have a man who, until welcome death reunites them, feels condemned to wander the world as an outsider in search of a missing complementary half.

Evidence

Before I revisit my opening conundrums in the light of the 'Schubert as single surviving twin' hypothesis, we should ask ourselves whether there is any evidence to support it. That some twins survive intra-uterine catastrophes which claim the life of their 'companion in the womb' is a matter of obstetric fact. Moreover there is abundant testimony in the literature of psychoanalysis and psychotherapy both that intra-uterine experience has a recognisable influence on many aspects of personality development and that simple regression techniques can elicit what seem to be verifiable memories of such events[23]. However, to assert the general principle that single surviving twins occur and may be affected by their pre-natal experiences is not sufficient to establish that this was in fact what happened in Schubert's case.

Nowadays, evidence of the death *in utero* of a twin foetus would come from routine medical procedures such as ultrasound scanning. Evidence of the

---

[23] See, for example, Piontelli A (1992) *From fetus to child – an observational and psychoanalytic study.* Tavistock/Routledge, London.

psychological consequences for the survivor would be found in personality testing and statistical correlation studies of child development and behaviour, as well as from the experience of the individual who might choose to undergo birth regression as a form of psychotherapy. However, direct evidence of these kinds is of course not available in the case of someone who died 172 years ago. I am not aware of any accounts of the obstetric details of Elizabeth Schubert's pregnancy or of Franz's birth. Neither should we naïvely read any significance into Schubert's choice of a French farce involving twin brothers separated at birth as the subject of his 1819 Singspiel '*Die Zwillingsbrüder*', even though its opening scene is based on a dactylic rhythm to whose possible significance I shall return shortly.

Directly accessible evidence being lacking, we must therefore first ask, 'What, at this distance of time, would constitute evidence? What would historical evidence for the "surviving twin" hypothesis *look* like – or, in the case of a long-dead musician, "*sound* like"?' It will have to be indirect, circumstantial. We shall have to content ourselves with inferences drawn from Schubert's life and art.

Hollywood scriptwriters tell us that a character's values are revealed by the choices he makes under pressure[24]. When the chips are down, does he choose the girl or the money? By the same token, a composer's artistic and creative hallmarks – his personal preferences in melody, rhythm, form and subject matter – as well as the patterns of his social relationships, represent the unconscious choices made under the influence of *internal* psychological pressure. All such choices are capable of more than one interpretation or explanation. The longing for death is hardly a uniquely Schubertian phenomenon in the middle of German Romanticism, and Schubert's own individual complexities cannot be made entirely to explain the broad thrust of a much larger cultural movement of which he was only part[25]. So the most we can ask of any hypothesis such as mine is this: 'Is it plausible? And if so, is it helpful? Interesting? Does it allow us to find some aspects of his work explicable rather than arbitrary? Does it add to our sense of the composer as a gifted individual touched by a unique configuration of human circumstance?'

Let's see.

The conundrums solved?

Schubert's emotional profundity, and his attitude to death

I see Schubert as a man whose creative imagination was infused by an abiding sense of loss and incompleteness which the relatively happy circumstances of his subsequent life were insufficient to outweigh; a man in whose music we can discern an intra-uterine memory of two becoming one and a longing – a *Sehnsucht* – for that one to become two again, even if death is what it takes to reunite them. We have a man who, for no reason that his life circumstances will explain, often portrayed himself in his art – *Winterreise* being the obvious example – as a lone outcast wandering in a hostile world. Heine's poem set as '*Der Doppelgänger*', in which a horrified onlooker recognises the face of a grief-stricken

[24] McKee R (1997) *Story*. Methuen, London.
[25] Graham Johnson: personal communication, 1999.

and shadowy stranger as his own double, might be an almost literal description of Schubert himself. Death would be the way home to a longed-for reunion with a long-lost 'other half'.

The dactyl rhythm

I think that Schubert's dactyl rhythm – that obsessive alternation between two-ness and one-ness – is an adult artist's transformed recollection of actual antenatal events, a nostalgic and compulsive 'search for the missing other half'. In the dactyl rhythm, I suggest, we hear Schubert unconsciously but insistently driven to reiterate, 'I was two, yet have become one.'

With this in mind, listen afresh to the song '*Der Tod und das Mädchen*', (D. 531, 1817). It opens with the piano establishing a dactylic 'Am I one or two?' ambivalence in the minor key. When the voice enters, it is unexpectedly and suddenly turbulent, almost panicky. This upheaval then gradually subsides, the dactyl transformed into a major key, leaving a sense of fulfilment, resolution and peace. I suggest that this sequence – the one/two ambiguity, the turbulence and panic, resolving into the tranquillity of death – is more than a flight of Romantic fancy. It is more than an allegory of Schubert's life, more than a metaphor, more than a symbol. I suggest it is a memory – non-verbal, pre-verbal, admittedly – but an artistic transformation nevertheless of real intra-uterine experience. I think that when Schubert writes music like this, he is expressing perceptions, impressions, conclusions which have been a part of him, quite literally, throughout his life. These feelings are so much at the core of him that I think he is communicating, quite literally, what it felt like to be inside his mother's womb and to have survived whatever tragedy took the life of his twin.

The 'volcanic outbursts'

The next time you listen to the A major piano sonata or the 9th symphony, and hear the flow of music unexpectedly engulfed in uproar and turbulence, ask yourself if it might not at some deep level be an actual memory given musical expression. Of the cataclysmic passage towards the end of the second movement of the C major symphony already referred to, Hugh Macdonald writes[26]:

> 'This most violent of passages ... is demonic, and of all climaxes in Schubert it is the only one which seeks and finds its own violent resolution, ... as though some great evil force had been exorcized.'

Listen to it – and see if it might not be the sound of your own twin miscarrying. If you buy into my interpretation, it is possible to hear the twins' mounting terror, a catastrophic death-blow, a numbed pause, then a dactylic realisation that one has survived and must carry on, the rest of life a burdensome delay until in 'easeful death' the surviving one becomes again the original two.

---

[26] Hugh Macdonald: *op. cit.*

His intense friendships

This side of the grave, however, the closest Schubert could come to that longed-for reunion was a succession of intense friendships. After leaving the family home, he moved from one Platonic liaison to another in a series of close and confiding, yet transient, 'best friend' relationships. Schubert's social life seems to have been a search, ultimately unfulfilled and incapable of fulfilment, for a Doppelgänger who, I suggest, was his unborn twin.

In conclusion

The artist is someone who can take pain and the commonplace and spin them into unforgettable insights. The hypothesis set out in this paper will, I know, antagonise some and be found ludicrous by others. Nevertheless, as a specialist in human complexity and a wide-eyed lover of Schubert's music, I find that to have some possible inkling of the ghosts that may have both inspired and haunted him makes 'the little mushroom' even more special.

Index